The
Bikini
Body
Diet

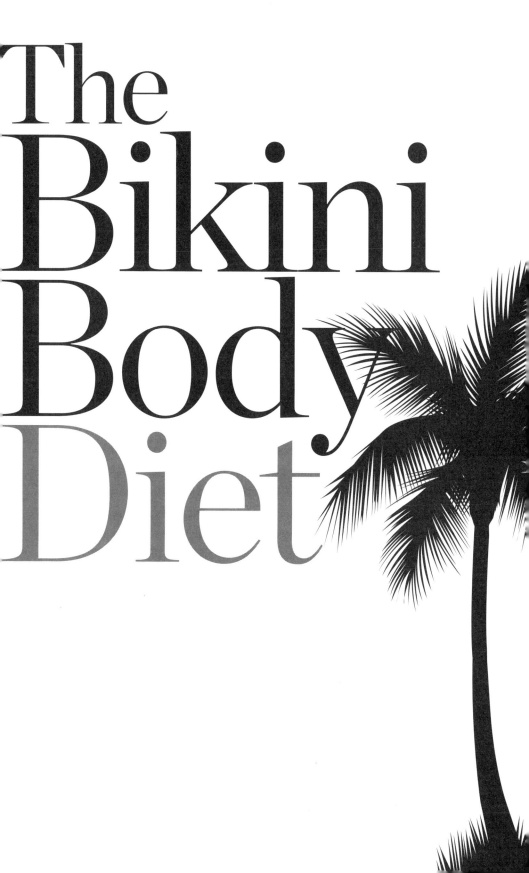

The Bikini Body Diet

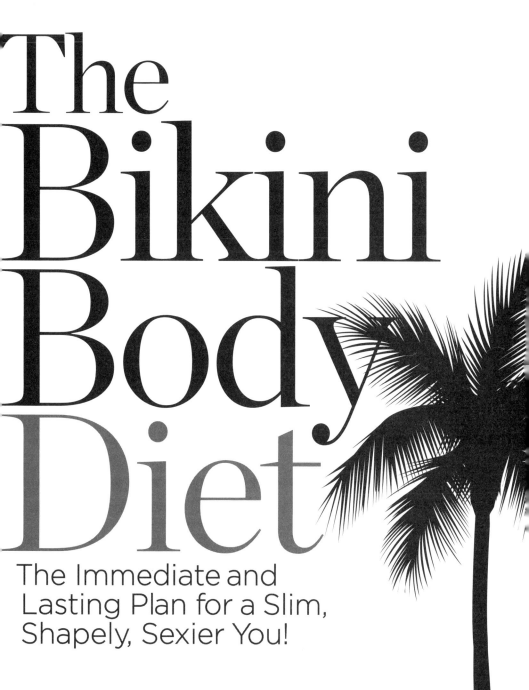

The Immediate and Lasting Plan for a Slim, Shapely, Sexier You!

By Tara Kraft
and the Editors of **SHAPE**

Foreword by David Zinczenko,
author of *Eat It to Beat It!*

No book can replace the diagnostic expertise
and medical advice of a trusted physician.
Please be certain to consult with your doctor before
making any decisions that affect your health,
particularly if you suffer from any medical condition or
have any symptom that may require treatment.

Published in the United States by
Galvanized Books,
a division of Galvanized Brands, LLC, New York

Galvanized Books is a trademark of
Galvanized Brands, LLC

ISBN 9780989594042

Printed in the United States of America on acid-free paper

2 4 6 8 9 7 5 3 1

Book design by George Karabotsos

Palm tree illustration by Heather Jones

GALVANIZED

To every woman who wants
to look and feel her best.

CONTENTS

CONTENTS

Acknowledgments

This book would not have been possible without the support of 12 million *Shape* readers, and the wise folks who helped shepherd this plan through, especially David Pecker, Chairman and CEO of American Media, Inc.; and David Zinczenko, President and CEO of Galvanized Brands, LLC.

Thanks also to my co-writers Ted Spiker and Sophie Knight; the staff of *Shape* magazine, especially deputy editor Jeanine Detz and contributing editor Candice Kumai; the team at American Media, Inc., especially Daniel Rotstein, Kevin Hyson, Dave Leckey, Steven Jacobs, June Steinfeld, Paula Buzzard, and Amanda Junker; Steve Perrine and George Karabotsos at Galvanized Brands; my colleagues at *Men's Fitness,* especially Brian Good and Cat Perry; and Libby Mcguire, Lisa Feuer, Mark Mcguire, Richard Callison, Nina Shields, Samantha Irwin, and the folks at Penguin Random House.

Foreword

By David Zinczenko
New York Times bestselling author of
Eat It to Beat It! and *The Abs Diet*

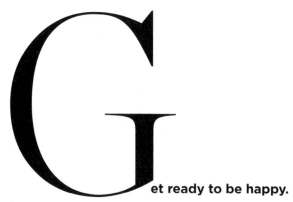

et ready to be happy.

How can I say that? Because I know what's in this book. It's exactly what you want: an express-lane pass to the body you've always wanted.

This book brings into focus the simple strategies you need to rediscover your best body ever, and keep it for life.

It's so easy to get lost these days: Lost in work, lost in social and family obligations, lost in the constant demands of our 24/8 society (wait...how many days in a week again?). When distractions happen, compromises happen. Surprise meeting at the office? Oh well, no noon workout. And the food at that meeting? Oh well, the fried dumplings will have to do.

Even your best intentions to make healthy choices can be sabotaged by a broken schedule, fatigue, or stress (or all three, as they tend to travel in packs like wolves). The convenience of processed food becomes a full-blown crutch. The occasional indulgence of a craving—because you deserve it—becomes habit.

Then, you put in for a vacation. You're looking for a beach or maybe a big boat surrounded by water. Heck, even a hotel pool will do. Somewhere warm. Somewhere sunny. Somewhere *else*.

And now you want to put on a bathing suit.

Or maybe you have a big date coming up—a reunion, a party, a lunch date with that ex who deserves to feel really bad that he broke up with you. And now you realize that all the lost workouts, lost meals, and lost time have left you with another loss: Your body confidence.

You know what? It's time to take it all back. It's time to reclaim your body and your life. It's time to start smiling again.

I've written a few books myself on healthy eating and exercise, and I'm here to tell you that the *Bikini Body Diet* delivers the goods in the fastest, simplest, most efficient, and foolproof way possible. Once you start the program, you'll be smiling. I know this because I know the people who run *Shape* magazine—the creators of the plan. Editor-in-chief Tara Kraft and her team have spent years analyzing everything from evolving nutritional science to the smart, simple tips that work in real life. And you know what? They know this program works—because many of them use it.

Another reason you'll be smiling: I know other women who have transformed themselves with the information in these pages, women who don't happen to work in the health and fitness field. They, too, have discovered how easy and effective the Bikini Body Diet is.

It isn't complicated. But it does need you. Without you, and your drive, and your commitment, it's just a bunch of ideas. Great ideas, to be sure. Scientifically proven, real-woman-tested ideas, you bet. But ideas without action leaves you with ... just the dream of what could be.

Stop dreaming. The Bikini Body Diet offers you an attainable goal: A lean, healthy, sexy body in just weeks. That alone will bring the smile back to your face.

And that smile will look as good on you as the swimsuit.

INTRODUCTION

Reveal Your Bikini Body

My name is Tara Kraft, editor-in-chief of *Shape* magazine. And I do not have a perfect bikini body.

But I like my body in a bikini or any bathing suit, for that matter. Why? I use the plan in this book, and I've learned to embrace the fun factor when it comes to how I view my body, especially when the weather gets warm and the beach calls me.

That's what I want for you. That's what this book is all about. Injecting some fun back into your life, helping you feel good about your body, projecting confidence and sex appeal, and doing it all with a great big smile.

Oh, and we'll do all this together in just six weeks.

As the editor-in-chief at *Shape,* it's my job to help all women build body confidence. Every month, every issue, I have to convince celebrities like Beyoncé, Britney Spears, Pink, and Jillian Michaels to pose in bikinis for the close inspection of millions of readers. Even the most famous, successful, and beautiful women in the world become nervous as 14-year-olds when confronted with the prospect of wearing a bikini.

So I know how daunting it is for us mere mortals. During a planning meeting for our 2012 swimsuit issue, my editors and I discussed the wide range of emotions that donning a swimsuit can trigger in women of all shapes and sizes:

From terror to pride...

From fear to joy...

From humility to bring it on...

Our cover model for that issue—Malin Ackerman—is the perfect example of what the ideal swimsuit shape is all about: a sleek, sexy body brimming with confidence. She's a gorgeous actress who eats well and admittedly possesses some terrific genes. But as a staff we didn't necessarily feel as confident about our own bodies as Malin seemed to be about hers. We went around the table and began sharing bathing suit burnouts.

Backing into pools wearing a cover-up... Trying on suits in crowded dressing rooms with unflattering lighting... Co-ed swim lessons in junior high! Any of these sound familiar?

All of a sudden the conversation turned: How could we, as a staff, rise to a body-confidence challenge, feel beautiful and strong, and put our words into action? And that's when my executive editor and fashion director had an idea that changed me, that changed the way I think about my body, and that inspired this book.

They wanted me to pose for the readers.

In a bikini.

(*Gulp*)

How great would it be, they argued, to show the editor-in-chief facing her body fears by stripping down and standing up?

In a panic, my mind flew to the recent late nights at the office, eating pizza at my desk while editing pages, and a winter of indulging in comfort food and red wine. We dropped the idea. (Being the boss helped sway my staff off the idea, believe me.)

But as a few weeks passed, I realized that as the face of a women's fitness and health magazine, I also had to be the body. I needed to be a role model for the women on my staff and for all my readers. I had to get out of my head, beat my insecurities, and face my fears about revealing my physique. It was very important that the whole experience feel real and organic and not like some publicity stunt. I wanted to do this because of everything it represented, everything it could represent.

The only catch: I had six weeks until the shoot.

Six weeks until I had to step in front of a camera and expose myself (quite literally) to 12 million potential critics (the harshest one being myself). Six weeks to get my body—and my mind—right. Would I do it? Could I do it?

I would. I could. I did.

And in just six weeks, you can, too.

Shapelier and Sexier in Just Six Weeks

The bikini, really, is the ultimate gut check.

We all have our ups and downs on the scale and hide under layers in winter months, but there's nothing you can hide in a swimsuit. And this is exactly why it stirs up so many emotions in women. We know the tricks and strategies to maximize our figures and to feel more confident, but the swimsuit strips all of us down to our body basics: How lean are we, how toned are we, how strong are we, how healthy are we?

And that's exactly why I wrote this book: I want all women not only to feel and look better in their bathing suits. I want them to feel stronger and be healthier. I don't want cover-ups to cover up. I don't want you to hide from feelings, from figuring out what can help you, from finding your best body. And above all, I want you to have fun!

When I sat down to devise my perfect (and, ahem, fear-based) six-week plan, the first thing I did was dive into the *Shape* archives and collect the smartest, most sensible, most scientifically proven tips and tricks we'd ever published. Believe me, nobody spends as much time thumbing through medical journals, nutrition news reports, and exercise research studies as we do. From the latest science, the ultimate superfast slim-down plan began to take shape.

But here's the trump card: I also did something even the top weight-management scientists can't do. I sought out the secrets of the women whose livelihoods depend on staying shapely and sexy. And when you have people like Jillian Michaels on speed dial; when Beyoncé is tearing it up in your photo studio, showing you her latest dance moves for a cover shoot; and when Britney Spears is donning yoga gear and demonstrating the belly-flattening moves right in front of you that got her bikini body back after two kids—well, let's just say a lot of researchers would jump to have access to these bodies of knowledge.

What I've learned is that while, yes, celebrities can often afford personal trainers, nutritionists, chefs, and other advantages that the rest of the population can't, the bottom line is that, in many ways, they deal with the same things we do. They have insane schedules. They have lots of people who demand their time. They want to look good. They're tempted by cheesecake. They don't work out eight hours a day. They're inse-

BIKINI BODY DIET SUCCESS!

Pamela Dropped Two Dress Sizes to Reveal Six-Pack Abs!

"My stomach was always a 'problem area.' Now, I can't stop staring at the definition on my tummy!" —*Pamela Makuta, Virginia*

Pamela has always been self-conscious about her midsection, and when people started asking if she was pregnant (she wasn't), she knew something had to give. Enter the Bikini Body Diet. Pamela shrank from a size 8 to a size 4 when she ditched a diet of processed foods, kicked caffeine to the curb, and swapped her gym-centric routine for a more flexible at-home regimen. "I always hated my stomach, but now I'm proud to look in the mirror. It's so flat!"

cure on the inside about how they look on the outside. And given the stakes, their insecurity often runs much deeper than yours or mine.

The major difference is that they're armed with knowledge that you may not have had access to. Until now. I've been to virtually every *Shape* bikini cover shoot for the past four years, and I've seen the mind-blowing results of these well-conceived diet and fitness strategies. And what I've learned is that it's totally doable to get that cover-model-worthy body. The Bikini Body Diet is about finding ways around your real-life challenges and giving you the information you need to make smart eating and exercise choices; it's about giving you the confidence to, yes, reveal all (or at least, *most!*).

Anybody can have a great body if they work out four hours a day or have perfect meals hand-delivered to them by a personal chef. But we at *Shape* know that life makes those things impossible.

But the Bikini Body Diet is all about the possibilities.

Little Tricks, Big Results

So how did I pull off my swimsuit photo shoot? In that six-week crunch beforehand, I had to de-bloat, tone, and crush my insecurity monster. And like you, I needed to get into the best shape of my life while going about my extremely busy life.

I pulled together all the success secrets I've learned along the way working at *Shape:* Tips from celebrities, my amazing fitness and nutrition teams, and most important, a world-renowned staff of expert advisors who helped supplement my own knowledge of what has worked wonders for *Shape* readers over the years. What woman wouldn't want a personal army like that to help her out?

Well, now that personal army is fighting for you. It is not some fad diet cooked up by food marketers. It is a guide of tried-and-tested techniques that help whittle your middle and make you feel gorgeous when it comes time for the big "reveal."

So...I had the perfect plan. I had the motivation. And then it was time for the shoot itself. How did it go?

Bodywise, I felt great that day. After following this plan, my stomach was flatter than it had ever been, my hips and thighs seemed sleeker, and when I moved, I could feel the strength I had developed. The only things that jiggled were the things I wanted jiggling! But as soon as I got to the studio, where I'd actually have to wear the bikini, I reverted to my junior-high self. I realized that this was not going to be as easy as I thought. Being in great shape isn't enough; you have to truly feel that you look your best.

I tried on dozens of suits in my office, behind closed doors, and the reality of what was taking place started to kick in. This was supposed to be fun? It wasn't. Then, as the pile of crumpled bikinis started to build around my feet, I finally found the one I felt wonderful in. It made me feel confident. It hugged me in all the right places, covered the areas I needed covered, and made me feel comfortable with my body. It was at that moment I decided to write this book, and I realized that it needed to be more than the ultimate weight-loss plan. That's why, you'll find whole chapters dedicated to grooming, fashion, and confidence building, so that you can fearlessly rock that bikini.

I walked to the set with a robe wrapped around me, and then, too quickly, it was time to begin. I dropped the robe and very shyly began posing for the camera. But then a funny thing happened. As the camera clicked away I started to channel my inner supermodel. I

BIKINI BODY DIET SUCCESS!

Tami Shed the Baby Weight— and Changed Her Life!

"I never would have dreamed I could look and feel this good!" —Tami Fisher, Arkansas

A busy mother of two young children, Tami never imagined she could get her pre-baby body back. But the flexible workout routines and healthy eating plan in the Bikini Body Diet transformed her figure—and her career goals! "I'm so inspired by the changes," Tami says, "I hope to transition into a health and fitness career!"

The Bikini Body Diet

thought about how motivated I was the past six weeks and all the times in my life I had tried to hide my body from the world instead of celebrating it.

Suddenly, with a crew of people staring at me in next to nothing, I felt an overwhelming sense of pride in myself. I felt strong and HOT and had a true appreciation for the skin I'm in.

I started having fun in a bathing suit again.

For the past two years, I've continued to use the Bikini Body Diet principles to keep myself in shape. It's my greatest wish that all of you have this same experience. With some work and lots of self-love, you can feel and look fabulous in bikinis, skinny jeans, sexy party dresses, and more. I am so excited for the journey you are about to embark on and look forward to seeing you proudly strutting your stuff.

Tara Kraft
Vice President/Editor-in-Chief
Shape magazine

INTRODUCTION

Bikini Body

Meals

3

per day,
no snacking

The 7-Day Super Slim-down

WEEK 1:
Two meals are homemade juices and one is a Bikini Body Diet recipe; cut out alcohol, sugars not found in fruit, added salt. You'll see incredibly fast results!

Bikini Body Diet Foods

Follow the BEACH rules:

BODY BUFFERS—
Muscle-building proteins

EVERYDAY ENERGIZERS—
Fruits (eat a serving at each meal)

ALL-U-CAN-EAT ANCHORS—
Vegetables (as much as you want)

CRUCIAL CARBS—
Good grains
(there are healthy ones)

HERBS AND SPICES—
Flavor enhancers

Cheat Sheet

Portion Size

All food portions the size of your fist, except vegetables

Plate Makeup

Half your plate with fruits and vegetables, other half with portioned proteins, fats, and healthy carbohydrates on the BEACH foods list

Liquids IN

Water, homemade juices, green tea, coffee, 1 glass of wine or clear alcohol a day, soup

Liquids OUT

Soda, diet soda, other sweetened juices or drinks

Cheat Meals

Once a week, after the 7-Day Super Slimdown

Extras

Add in supplements of magnesium and vitamin D

Bikini Body Diet Workout

HIGHER INTENSITY CIRCUITS, focusing on bikini-baring body parts, such as **LEGS** and **BUTT**.

HIGH-INTENSITY INTERVAL TRAINING for cardio to **BURN FAT.**

CHAPTER 1

The Right Way to Eat

Better Foods for a Better Body

I **hope you're ready for fast and permanent changes.**
On this plan, you're going to be able to change your body in terms
of pounds, inches, and the way you feel. And you'll notice those changes
right away—in the very first week. Best of all, the benefits just keep on
coming. Follow the Bikini Body Diet and you'll experience all kinds of
life changes—changes that will improve and enrich your life all year-
round, and for years to come.

1

The Bikini Body Diet

Here's a sampling:

You'll lose inches from your waist. By eating the Bikini Body Diet foods in smart but satisfying portions, you'll keep your metabolism revving, searching for body fat to burn—and going right for that hard-to-banish belly fat. (And you'll target belly fat even more with our additional workout plans.)

You'll trim and tone those bikini-baring body parts, like your butt, thighs, and hips. As the extra flab melts away, you'll begin to add in special trouble-zone-toning exercises, giving your body a double-whammy: Those body parts will firm up and slim down at the same time. Plus, as you reduce some water retention with our plan, you'll achieve an even slimmer look (not to mention feel better).

You'll be happier. And peppier. The ingredients and foods that are the focus of the Bikini Body Diet have been shown to improve mood and increase long-term energy. Rather than allowing you to fall into the all-too-common energy slumps associated with our busy schedules and blood-sugar-spiking diets, this plan gives you the tools to feel better all-around, which then inspires you to do better and better, which further bolsters your mood and energy. A vicious cycle—without the vicious part!

Uno's Personal Deep Dish Cheese Pizza
2,310 calories

YOU ATE IT? NEGATE IT!
3 hours of jumping rope

You'll sleep better and get more done. Not only will the diet and exercise plans in this book help improve your sleep habits, but the natural supplements that are part of this program have been shown to improve sleep and stabilize your circadian rhythm. (And by the way—sleep is critical to maintaining your weight! You'll learn why in the pages to come.)

You'll reduce the risks of some of the most serious diseases and conditions that a woman faces, including high blood pressure, heart disease, diabetes, cancer, and stroke. I'll outline the science later in the book, but numerous studies show that the power-packed nutrients that are emphasized in the Bikini Body Diet are some of nature's best disease-fighters.

2

And perhaps most important of all, you'll look and feel more confident in your clothes, out of your clothes, and yes, even in a bikini. As a woman, a mother, a friend, a lover, a worker—every aspect of your life will improve as you feel your sense of accomplishment grow. Over the years, *Shape* readers have reported that losing weight has changed their lives. They've become more adventurous. They've become better people. They've gone from needing to be inspired to becoming the inspiration.

You're going to achieve all of these things with a sensible, smart, and healthy six-week eating and exercise plan that will give you results you can feel—and show off—in just the first few days. (That's how effective the 7-Day Super Slimdown is.) And you'll learn terrific secrets of weight-loss science (for example, the one kind of grain that's been shown to change your body composition to reduce the size of your middle! Who says you shouldn't eat carbs?).

Plus, it's about as easy as it gets. No crazy formulas, no counting or measuring or logging, no algebra or calculus to tell you when you're allowed to have a carb. Very quickly, you're going to learn the foods that will make you lean, then follow a few simple guidelines for how and when to eat them to trigger your body's natural fat burners—setting you on the fast track to losing pounds and inches.

What you may find most appealing about this plan is that it's going to give you the kick-start you need—and want. You'll see and feel results— as much as 5 to 7 pounds in just the first week— results that will inspire you to stick to the plan and reap all the rewards. And, if you so choose, you can add in a workout approach that will have your body primed for the beach (or a wedding or the bedroom or just showing off in all areas of life). By targeting those bikini-baring body parts, you will feel and look more toned than ever before.

BIKINI BODY DIET SUCCESS!

Nancy Transformed from Blasé to Bombshell!

"I dedicated myself to the Bikini Body Diet workouts and watched 10 pounds melt off my body!"
—Nancy Byers, Kansas

Being healthy and toned was Nancy's goal, but at 47, her body wasn't responding like it used to. The Bikini Body Diet was just what she needed to ignite her metabolism and sculpt lean, sexy curves in just six weeks. "I knew I needed to kick it up a notch. This was just the thing!"

So let's get right to it.

To go out into the world in a bikini, you have to strip down to the point where everything's exposed. At which point, everyone looks. That can be part of the fun and part of the terror. But here's a useful idea: Why should we be the only ones to go through that scrutiny? In this chapter, I want to strip something else down and force it—chubby bits and all—into the sunlight for all of us to inspect. I'm talking about the diet industry.

Being the editor-in-chief of *Shape,* I am part of the industry, so my goal here isn't to be hypocritical, or rip apart various plans and programs, because the truth is that many approaches can work, depending on the plan, depending on the woman, depending on lots of factors. But some of the principles that can work in theory may also backfire by actually negating some of the good things you may already be doing.

Most plans have pitfalls. You've probably hit them before. Well, I don't want you to hit them again. Part of the trick of embracing a diet plan is knowing where those pitfalls are dug in so you can gracefully hop over. That's why I love the Bikini Body Diet approach so much, and why it worked for me and for so many of the people who have tried it: It gives you the power and energy to succeed in those tricky moments where sticking to your weight-loss goals can become challenging. We do that from Week 1—starting with the 7-Day Super Slimdown—but then give you the tools in the form of BEACH foods to help you make smart choices no matter where you are, no matter what your schedule is, and no matter whether your personality drives you to want freestyle improvisation or stick-to-it rules.

So now, let's take a look at some of the major problems that many women are facing in the current state of dieting and weight-loss programs—and how the Bikini Body Diet helps address them.

PITFALL: The Healthy Food Trap

These days, many dieting trends are centered around making sure you get enough healthy foods and eliminate as many artificial or processed foods as possible. Eat from the earth; don't eat anything in a package. Meat, nuts, and greens good; pasta bad. In a lot of ways, that's absolutely appropriate and a smart approach to eating. Few people question the fact that we're better off eating fruits and vegetables than we are eating "muffins" that are jammed with more sugar than you'll find in a kindergarten class lost in Willy Wonka's chocolate factory. That's the basis for any good eating plan, and it's the basis for the Bikini Body Diet, too.

So what's the problem?

Many people—whether a diet plan calls for it or not—equate eating healthy food with eating *lots* and *lots* of healthy food. If it's good for me, there's no reason I can't have a zillion pieces! If it's natural, there are no limits! Chicken breasts to the ceiling!

So what happens? We get sold foods that sound healthy—especially in restaurants—and we help ourselves, without stopping to figure out what we're really eating. And the truth can be pretty crazy. Check out these good-sounding diet disasters:

P.F. Chang's Gluten-Free Fried Rice (must be healthy—it's gluten-free!): 1,360 calories, or a full day's worth for a woman

Sbarro Gourmet Spinach and Broccoli Pizza (oh, come on, it's spinach and broccoli!): 1,440 calories for two slices

California Pizza Kitchen Waldorf Salad (salad is good for you, right?): 1,290 calories per entrée

We'd all be better off if restaurants just told us we were eating junk, because we (quite logically) tend to overeat when we perceive something to be healthy. A study published in the *Journal of Consumer Research*

reported that people who dined at restaurants that claim to be healthy underestimate how many calories they consume by 44 percent. Kind of scary, right? Something in our brain tells us that if we're eating something we think is good, then it doesn't matter how much we have.

And over time, too much of any food—good or bad—can be stored as fat if not used for another function in the body.

So while the goal of eating natural and healthful food sounds smart, we have to be careful not to let our brains override basic biology: that too much of anything isn't a good thing.

The Bikini Body Diet Solution: By sticking to three meals a day and ball-parking your portion sizes to keep them reasonable (nobody has time for scales and measures!), you can help limit the excess calories you may be prone to eating, even in healthy foods. You will still eat healthily; after all, that's what the BEACH foods are all about. And you'll also eat them in balance, to help keep your satisfaction up and your appetite down.

Read a Nutrition Label Like a Pro

Reading the fine print on packaged foods can seem easy enough. That is, until you realize that half the words on it sound like they've come straight out of a science-fiction movie. While a government survey shows that most of us use nutrition labels to make choices, you have to know what you're actually reading. Some things to look out for:

✳ **Look at serving size.** "Serving size" doesn't always mean one package, even if that package is the size of your pinkie. Though it may be logical to think that one serving size would be a whole bottle, bag, or box (or muffin, as the case may be), you always have to do a quick calculation. Let's say you plan on

PITFALL: The Marketing of "Healthy" Food

There are many clear black-and-white areas when it comes to food choices. Broccoli good. Nacho cheese *gooood*, but really, really bad. Most of us know the difference (and the issue becomes whether we make the choice to avoid the temptation, not whether we know what's bad for us).

The food industry wants us to see GRAY. That's how they sell things. Food marketers want us to think that their food is doing something good for us, even if it's not. Nonfat foods can be loaded with sugar. And low-sugar foods can be loaded with tons of otherworldly gunk to help make them taste better.

Brilliant marketing tactics, of course. For the folks who desperately want to eat healthily but still crave cookies, these foods can serve as some sort of "feel-good" food. "I know I'm eating well because the box says I am!" So what's the harm in eating a box of all-natural cookies?! Turns out, quite a lot.

Starbucks grande salted caramel hot chocolate with whipped cream
640 calories

YOU ATE IT? NEGATE IT!

62 minutes on a stairclimber

---

drinking the whole bottle of chocolate milk and see, wow, it's only 100 calories! So you drink it. Only problem? That bottle is 2.5 servings, or 250 calories. Be sure you see the big picture (total fat, sodium, etc.), not just the calorie count.

✳ **Don't assume "reduced" means "none" or "low."** And in fact, the food could have high levels of sugar, sodium, or anything else—just that it's less than the full version. Other foods—especially baked goods and yogurts—love to advertise "low fat" or "fat free" though they've been packed with sugar. So look at the numbers, not the marketing lingo on the front.

✳ **Scan the ingredient list.** Good rule of thumb: The fewer ingredients, the better. If the list of ingredients would rival a Tolstoy work, look elsewhere. And make sure that sodium and sugars are as low as possible on that list (or better yet, not even on it).

7

Applebee's
Grilled
Chicken
Caesar
Salad
1,010 calories

YOU ATE IT?
NEGATE IT!
5 hours of
surfing

While there are certainly some products that are less evil than others, it points to an important Bikini Body Diet lesson: You can't trust the lingo; you have to look at the labels.

That's where the real story takes place: Where you'll see how the numbers (such as calories and fat grams) stack up per serving, which, by the way, is also an important number. Something may seem as if it's low-calorie, but if you examine how many servings come in a typical jar, box, or package, that can change the story dramatically. The labels also tell you whether sugar (and all its relatives) are packed high on the ingredient list. Bottom line: All the answers are in the fine print on the back, not on the big, colorful banners in large print on the front.

The Bikini Body Diet Solution: By basing most of your meals around our BEACH foods (and some of our delicious recipes, starting on page 90), you're going to avoid the traps that many fall into. But for times when you do buy pre-packaged foods, you must have a critical eye toward marketing jargon and examine the nutritional labels. Ultimately, you want foods low in sugar and with few ingredients (and as few artificial ones as possible). See the box on page 6 for tips on how to read a food label.

PITFALL: Calorie Counting As King

Many successful weight-loss plans revolve around one practice: Count everything. Log everything. Hold yourself accountable for every single thing that travels through your mouth. And do not go over a certain calorie number every day. If you do? MAJOR FAIL!

Now, don't misunderstand: There can be tremendous benefits from this kind of accountability. Many people, including many of the readers of *Shape*, have had success using some variation of the calorie-counting method. And if it works for you, that's wonderful. It can be a fine way, especially, to get a plan going and to examine how much food you're really eating (and how much of it's unnecessary). It does help you feel accountable and learn which foods are generally high in calories and which are not, so you can make better eating choices and figure out what foods will keep you fuller for the

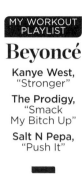

MY WORKOUT PLAYLIST

Beyoncé

Kanye West, "Stronger"

The Prodigy, "Smack My Bitch Up"

Salt N Pepa, "Push It"

Your Guide to Eating Out

You don't need to ditch the Bikini Body Diet principles just because you're eating out. Yes, restaurants can make it very hard to stay true to the principles I've outlined here, but that doesn't mean you have to sacrifice taste. If you do have a feel-good meal that you look forward to and want to indulge in, then save it for your cheat meal and enjoy, but other times, you can navigate the tricky waters of the restaurant world with a few strategies.

✴ **Employ your same plate principles—lean meats, vegetables, and healthy carbs.** No healthy carb options on the menu? Ask for a double-dose of vegetables, or order a baked potato, scoop out most of the inside, and eat the tasty skin.

✴ **Send the bread back.** Ask if you can have some raw vegetables instead. Or order a cup of soup, or salad with dressing on the side, to get you going.

✴ **Tell your server you don't want any extra butter.** Restaurants are known for sloshing it on everything from vegetables to steaks to give their foods more glow (and taste). Make it clear you don't want the extra.

✴ **Say that you have dietary restrictions.** Request a piece of chicken or fish with steamed vegetables, and encourage the chef to have fun with the spices. Oftentimes, they'll find it refreshing to create a new concoction or you.

✴ **Take half and box it up before you start.** It's a great way to create a waistline-friendly meal. Plus you'll save money—leftovers can be a tasty lunch the next day!

✴ **Order your glass of wine toward the end of your meal;** that way, the sweetness can go with dinner, but also act as a low-cal dessert.

Ashley Made the Junk Food Disappear!

"I usually give in to temptation, but this made it so easy to stay strong!"
—*Ashley McCann, Illinois*

Ashley had tried every diet out there but could never fully commit. Yet junk-food temptations were no match for the Bikini Body Diet. Dropping an easy five pounds while enjoying delicious, satisfying meals was just what Ashley needed to stay on track. "I can't wait to keep progressing on the program. I would absolutely recommend this to all of my girlfriends."

fewest calories (one important way that vegetables play a role).

Over the long term, though, calorie counting can be a tough way to sustain weight loss. In fact, it can even backfire. While apps and other digital toys have made it much easier to track calories, it can also be hard to maintain for those of us (all of us!) with busy lifestyles. And lastly, the one thing that counting calories won't do is to ensure that you're getting the right *types* of calories. On a 1,200-calorie-a-day diet, well, six glasses of wine and half a burger sounds like a fine day! But that's not optimal for nutrition, health, energy levels, and so many other things.

While that may be an extreme example, calorie counting can promote that kind of behavior—very few calories throughout the day and a splurge-fest on a pepperoni platter during happy hour. There may be nothing wrong with that approach every once in a while, but it can quickly become a ritual—one that sounds good ("I'm sticking under my calorie count!"), but really isn't.

The Bikini Body Diet Solution: Once you pick your BEACH foods or recipes, nearly every portion on your plate should be about the size of your fist (*your* fist, not the Hulk's). Few people have time for scales and strict measuring, but the fist test is a very good approximation of a typical serving. This approach—of controlling portions of healthy foods—allows you to have nutritional balance at a reasonable quantity. (You can go over fist-size on some foods, like vegetables, when prepared healthily. Feel free to eyeball those portions at the size of a Prius.)

PITFALL: Compensation Eating

**Mandy
Moore**

I see it all the time. Heck, I even feel it a lot. After an especially tough workout, you feel good. You feel strong. You feel happy. You feel energized. You also feel like eating your laptop because you're so hungry. So what happens? You rationalize. "I worked out hard, so hard that I am certain I have burned one gazillion calories. I shall have the three-foot long club. With mayo. And I shall still lose weight!" A study published in the journal *Appetite* found that people who were told to visualize working out reached for up to 60 percent more snack food than those who weren't told to contemplate going to the gym.

Cass Elliot,
"California
Earthquake"

Yellow,
"Don't Bring
Me Down"

**Fleetwood
Mac,**
"Secondhand
News"

**The Bird and
the Bee,**
"Polite Dance
Song"

Neil Finn,
"Driving Me
Mad"

It's a normal and natural reaction. While there are some athletes who burn enough calories to justify these huge compensation servings, the reality is that most of us do not. Even if you're going hard for an hour, you may be burning only 500 or 600 calories, and that's certainly not enough to justify seconds or doing a triple-loop through the buffet line.

The Bikini Body Diet Solution: The workouts here (starting on page 111) will help you burn fat and tone your trouble zones. But they're not the kind of workouts that will leave you so famished that you want to clear out a pancake house. It's also important to remember that sometimes these hunger cues are really thirst cues, so making sure you're properly hydrated can help decrease the hunger pangs you may experience with exercise. And in a pinch, you can also reach for one of our special juices or soups to help satisfy your cravings without taking a huge caloric toll on your body.

PITFALL: Mini-Meals

Very recently, we've seen a shift in diet thinking: Lots of people are pushing the mini-meal approach. Eat five to eight times a day to keep the metabolism roaring, but just make them small meals. Only problem? Lots of people subscribe to the "five to eight times a day," but not so much to the "small" meals.

MY WORKOUT PLAYLIST

Marisa Tomei

Edward Sharpe & The Magnetic Zeros, "Up from Below"

Machito, "Kenya"

Dead Man's Bones, "Dead Man's Bones"

Patsy Cline, *Patsy Cline Golden Hits*

Frank Sinatra, *The Capitol Years*

One study from Purdue University found that mini-meals may be flawed because people underreport their calories. Think about it: To make a six-meal-a-day strategy work, most of your meals and snacks would have to be in that 200- to 300-calorie limit. While not so difficult to do for, say, a mid-morning snack, that's generally not happening for lunch, dinner, and probably even breakfast. So add up all the caloric overload, and those six or seven meals quickly have the look of a very high-calorie day.

Now, this "grazing" approach can work, but I generally see it working only if you're one of the few people who are really good about sticking to those strict measuring and counting practices.

The Bikini Body Diet Solution: Your three meals, packed with BEACH foods, will keep you satisfied and your energy high. And most importantly, they'll keep you from overeating by allowing you to feel some wiggle room with snacks. Some people do feel the need to eat a little more or crave something late at night, so during those times, I'd encourage you to reach for one of our special juices—they can satisfy sweet cravings and help keep hunger down, especially in times when your body feels as if it needs a little extra kick.

CHAPTER 2

Bring On the Bikini Body!

The 6 Sexy Secrets!

The following six principles are the backbone of the Bikini Body Diet plan, the overriding guidelines that will show you how to eat and exercise. The details are included here, as well as throughout the book, but the umbrella principles are what this program is all about—eating smart, getting strong, and feeling sexy.

SEXY STRATEGY #1:

Treat Yourself to the 7-Day Super Slimdown

Visualize this: You're wrapped in a fluffy, white, warm towel, with soothing music in the background, a candle, the smell of your favorite aromas. Maybe lavender or vanilla or peppermint. Your mind and body have melted into the serenity of your favorite spa treatment. A massage, a pedi, a facial, a scrub... While they all have their own purposes, there's a common element to most of these kinds of pampering treatments. They're not just about relaxation; they're about rejuvenation: Exfoliating the dry skin, flushing toxins from your body, or just plain making you full of life and energy.

Sexy Strategy #1 is about giving your insides the same kind of treatment. It's pretty similar to the way we do it for our outsides—we get rid of the nasty stuff to let the good things work their magic.

That's what the 7-Day Super Slimdown will do: Rejuvenate you nutritionally—with significant effects in both the short term (up to 2 ½ inches lost from your waist) and in the long term as you embrace the eating principles of the diet.

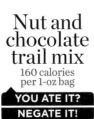

Nut and chocolate trail mix
160 calories per 1-oz bag

YOU ATE IT?
NEGATE IT!

17 minutes of jumping jacks

So the major kick-starter on the Bikini Body Diet is to take the first week and pamper your insides. Full disclosure: It may not always be easy, especially if you haven't paid attention to your eating habits in quite some time (massages can hurt, after all, but the dividends are worth it, no?). But what it will do is give you the jump that you need. Why? Because you'll flush your body of any of the bad things you've been pumping into it, and you'll also reduce bloat and any extra water you may be retaining.

But make no mistake, this is no cleanse in the wipe-the-pipes-of-everything-and-anything sense. This is about getting back to basics and filling your body with rich, healthy nutrients that will not only give you energy but also give your body a much-needed internal scrubbing.

Diets succeed only if they're flexible; you have to adapt what you eat to how you live. But for the first week—*and just for one week!*—you're going to follow a strict regimen. If you do, you will see your body change right before your eyes, and it will give you the motivation you need to follow this diet's overall guidelines and get the body you want.

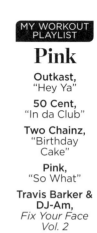

MY WORKOUT PLAYLIST

Pink

Outkast, "Hey Ya"

50 Cent, "In da Club"

Two Chainz, "Birthday Cake"

Pink, "So What"

Travis Barker & DJ-Am, *Fix Your Face Vol. 2*

Pick your start day, do your food shopping (recipes start on page 90), and get ready to hunker down. For. Just. One. Week.

The rules:

Cut all alcohol. Though there's a time and a place for it, booze gives you calories you don't need right now (not to mention the fact that it can lower inhibitions and increase junk-food cravings and overeating). There will be plenty of booze cruises for you to enjoy once you're into that swimsuit. For now, let's take a week to be super-healthy.

Cut any extra sodium. You'll do this naturally just by keeping to the food rules that follow, but do not add extra salt to your meals. Nearly 90 percent of people consume more than the recommended 2,300 milligrams a day. (Salt causes water to move from your bloodstream into your skin, which is why a dose of cheese puffs will give you a *puffy* look.) The good part about cutting sodium is that while you're looking better, you'll also be getting healthier. A study in the *American Journal of Clinical Nutrition* found that even a single salty meal can do damage in just half an hour. The reason? Sodium may interfere with one of the chemical processes that helps your blood vessels expand, meaning it's easier for cholesterol to stick to your arteries.

Cut the sugar. No desserts. No sugars not naturally found in the BEACH foods or in our recipes. So yes, fruits are fine; Fruity Pebbles are not. (Don't panic. This is for seven days only. There are plenty of decadent desserts in the days to follow—you'll find some delicious samples starting on page 107.)

Have only three meals every day. No grazing, no "eat every two hours." That's been the nutrition fad of the past few years, but as discussed in detail earlier, the latest research suggests that having more meals only leads to increased calorie consumption—even though you're trying to keep the numbers down.

Have two Bikini Body Diet juices—one for breakfast, one for lunch—for each of the first seven days. Then have one of our recipes for dinner. While the calories may be lower than what you're eating right now, these three meals have enough nutrition to power you throughout your day. This is not about starving, which, in the end, only drives you to want to eat more. Instead, you'll be establishing a pattern of basing your meals on fruits and vegetables. You'll also find that a healthy juice (not one packed with sweeteners) can help keep you satisfied long enough to get

Sneaky Secrets for Better Eating

THE STRATEGIES in this chapter give you the overarching principles for how to get your best bikini body. Sometimes, though, you may need a little help putting them into action. These tricks can help you do just that.

Pick your favorite recipes and rotate them. According to research published in the *American Journal of Clinical Nutrition,* women who were served the same meal for five consecutive days consumed less by the end of the week, while those who ate the same meal once a week for five weeks ending up eating more calories. The point: You'll be better off choosing a few favorites and eating them over and over, rather than always trying to come up with new ways to satisfy your taste buds. Also, it suggests that the best way to make our meals is by making enough to have leftovers. Tip: As soon as you're done making it, put the left-

you to your next meal. In many ways, it's the perfect way to have a quick, nutrient-packed meal on the go as you start your day, or if find yourself swamped in the middle of a hectic one.

Make time in your schedule for the Bikini Body Diet workouts. These workouts will challenge your heart and muscles by combining cardiovascular exercise with resistance training. Studies show that a combination of cardio and light weights torches fat in three ways: during your workout; for 24 to 48 hours after your workout (the "afterburn" effect of a heightened metabolism); and for years to come, as you build permanent calorie-consuming lean muscle tissue that hungrily melts your problem areas. (More on these workouts in a moment.)

That's it. Pretty straightforward slimdown, wouldn't you say? Three daily meals, all detailed in the book, so there's no thinking, no worrying, no starving. Give yourself one week like this and then you'll use that as a foundation for your new eating habits. That's when you let the rest of the principles kick in. While this plan is a six-week program and you'll be

overs away so you're not tempted to go back for seconds.

Think about tomorrow. Scientists from Penn State and Texas A&M University found that people who focused on positive thoughts about the future were more likely to choose fruit over candy (as opposed to people who thought about the past).

Stop multitasking during meals. In a study from the University of Birmingham, people who read a newspaper while eating consumed more calories than those who listened to an audio track telling them to focus on food. When you're distracted, you're

likely to eat more. Enjoy your food, think about it, love it. Then move on to whatever's next at hand.

Play mind games. The foods in this plan are so packed with nutrients that it might sometimes feel like you're eating decadently, and that's a good thing. It's to your benefit to tell yourself that. A study in the journal *Health Psychology* found that people who thought they were drinking a higher calorie drink (even though they weren't) saw a steep decline in ghrelin (the hunger hormone) than those who thought the same drink had fewer calories.

this strict only during the first week, you can always use the 7-Day Super Slimdown as you need it—when you hit plateaus or feel you need a little jump-start to recover from an overindulgent weekend.

Turn Down the Volume

If we had to boil all of our body problems down to one sentence, most people in the health-care industry (and the general public) would use the same four words to identify the major culprit:

We eat too much.

No secret there, right? Our American restaurant portions are huge—they are practically large enough to feed an elephant. We have appetizers that have quadruple-digit calorie counts. We order drinks that should be dessert. At home or elsewhere, we snack far too often. We eat and eat and eat.

So our second strategy comes down to a very simple principle, though a little harder to follow if you're out of practice: No grazing.

Few of us can really stick to so-called small snacks. One hundred calories quickly becomes 200, which quickly becomes 300, which quickly becomes "Well, now I have to eat the entire row of cookies, you know, so the pack is even." And for most women, one of these snacks can make a huge dent in the amount you should be eating every day, which is about 1,200 calories. It takes 3,500 calories to build a pound of fat. If you're munching on a 200-calorie snack every day—that's half of a bagel or a handful of Gummy Bears—you can expect to gain a little more than 20 pounds in a single year. (As a general rule, every 100 calories you add a day is worth 10 pounds of yearly weight gain.) So in this plan, we're eliminating snacking (though we do make room for emergencies

Honey-roasted peanuts
250 calories per 1.38-oz bag

YOU ATE IT?
NEGATE IT!

31 minutes of jogging

as you go through the plan; more on page 94).

"But what about grazing on healthy foods?" you ask.

Even grazing on relatively healthy choices, like carrot sticks and hummus, can set us up for poor results. Consider this 2012 study in the journal *Nutrition & Diabetes*. Researchers measured the levels of serum carotenoid concentrations (a marker of increased fruit and vegetable consumption) between two groups trying to lose weight. One group increased fruit and vegetable consumption, while the other reduced calories. In the end, both groups increased their intake of fruits and vegetables (a good thing), but the group that cut calories lost more weight. Not a surprise, right? We gain when we eat more calories than we can burn up. Most studies showing people losing weight when eating six times a day were done under very controlled circumstances. Does "controlled circumstances" describe your life? Nope, mine either. The real-world danger that a multi-meal and multi-snack approach to daily eating is that we're simply more susceptible (except for the very, very strictest of us who have the patience to weigh, measure, and count everything) to going over our daily calorie goals when we give ourselves six opportunities to eat, as opposed to the traditional three.

Besides the obvious downside of increased calories that come from snacking, there are other negatives. A Japanese study, for example, found that nighttime snacking increased LDL cholesterol and decreased fat oxidation, which researchers suggested can change the metabolism of fat and increase the risk of obesity.

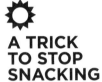

A TRICK TO STOP SNACKING

One of the big adjustments you may have to make, depending on your current eating style and frequency, is eliminating the tendency to snack every time you're bored or get a little pang in your belly. Fill your three meals with a good mix of BEACH foods to help keep you satiated and avoid those cravings. But there's nothing wrong with trying some other tricks, too. In a study from the University of Southern California, participants were given popcorn to eat while watching a movie. They were also told which hand to use to eat it. Those who used their non-dominant hand ate 30 percent less popcorn than those who didn't. The theory goes: The trick slows you down, so that not only may your full-feeling signals kick in, but you'll also realize that that the food you're eating is potentially bad for you.

The Bikini Body Diet

And a review of studies in the *American Journal of Clinical Nutrition* found eating six meals a day provided no weight-loss advantage. But as I said, when you eat six times a day, you're simply more likely to overeat and not have the same number of calories you would if you were eating three times a day.

Also, it seems as if there may be another advantage to sticking to the three squares: A 2012 University of Missouri study found that women who ate three meals a day had lower fat in their blood than those who ate six, even with the same total daily calories. (Important note: Eating three meals a day means eating three meals a day, not skipping some if you're on the go, or trying to save a few extra calories by skipping breakfast or working through lunch. According to research from the Fred Hutchinson Research Center in Seattle, dieters who skipped meals lost eight fewer pounds than those who ate three times a day.)

But there's another element to controlling volume. It's not just about the number of times you eat during the day: It doesn't do you a lick of good to reduce your meals/snack number from six to three if those three meals could feed a family of six.

So, in addition to knowing the foods you should center your meals around, you need to familiarize yourself with what a "serving" really looks like. Nowadays, when we have 2,000-calorie "personal" pizzas, it's easy to forget that a proper serving size of just about anything is about the size of your fist. The foods you'll eat will be easy enough to learn (look at Sexy Strategy #3), but portion control is the other important factor. Use these two guidelines to help steer you to healthy portions:

One, fill your plate just about halfway with fruits and vegetables and the other half with healthy proteins and healthy carbohydrates.

Two, keep each portion of the non-fruits-and-vegetables about the size of your fist. It's a simple eyeball test. And while it certainly gives you some room to cheat if you're so inclined ("Well, tonight, I'm going to use Sasquatch's fist as my guide"), the point is that it teaches you to develop an instinct—and consistent behavior—for eating proper portions

You don't need to stay in any magical "zone" or find a golden mean between fats, carbs, and protein. A study from the Pennington Biomedical Research Center in Louisiana studied four different diet strategies where the percentages of protein, fat, and carbs all varied. Over a two-year period, they all lost about the same amount of weight.

The payoff for keeping portion size under control, no doubt, is huge. In a Cornell University study, those people who ate smallish portions at lunch consumed nearly 250 fewer calories daily and lost a little more than a pound a week. This flies in the face of conventional wisdom, which tells you that if you eat small during the day, you'll gorge at night. Researchers say that after every meal your body resets itself, so smaller portions now won't make you gnaw the arm off your couch later, and you'll experience the benefits of fewer total calories consumed. Trust me, portion control works. I have a small soup for lunch every day—and I'm slimmer than I've ever been.

1 cup
potato
salad
358 calories

YOU ATE IT?
NEGATE IT!
62 minutes
of playing
softball

Finding balance in how you build your breakfast, lunch, and dinner plate has a great psychological effect, too: Research from Arizona State University found that people who cut up bagels into four pieces ate less of it than those who ate it whole. The effect lasted through their next meal, where the bite-size group consumed 40 percent fewer calories. The message: Small portions are a signal that can help you eat less. And a fist size roughly equates to the standard one-serving size of these foods, such as a four-ounce piece of chicken or fish, or a serving of whole-grain rice.

If you're a grazer or a big-meal eater, this approach will take some getting used to, but the 7-Day Super Slimdown will initially help you adjust to eating in a different way. And in a week or two after that, this will feel natural (and delicious!). So once you reach Week 2 the instructions are straightforward:

➤ Have three meals a day.

➤ Cover at least half your plate with fruits and veggies.

➤ Make portions the size of your fist for other foods.

SEXY STRATEGY #3:

Feast on BEACH Foods

Some diets call for strict eating plans—eat this, eat that, with no wiggle room. Other diets give you so much flexibility that you hit a slippery slope—into a tub of brownie batter. What I believe is the most effective eating strategy lies right in the middle: You have to have some guidelines, but within those, you also have some flexibility. You have to be able to know the parameters, but also know how to mix things up so that when you're faced with certain situations that can quickly spin out of your control (parties, happy hour, travel), you can adjust your eating accordingly. That's where the magic lies when it comes to losing weight: Have a system in place that is clear and smart but also considers, well, that life happens.

That's why I've developed an eating acronym that will help steer you in the right direction no matter your situation. All you have to remember is this: BEACH. If you make your meals center around these BEACH foods (also considering the previous principles of three meals and portion sizes), you're going to take in a healthy, nutrient-filled diet that's designed to make you lose fat and firm up. Now, when I say BEACH foods, you can safely assume I'm not talking about hot dogs and fries (though wait until you get a load of our pizza recipe). BEACH is the path to your best body:

MY WORKOUT PLAYLIST

Molly Sims

Rihanna,
"S&M"

Jay-Z featuring
Alicia Keys,
"Empire State
of Mind"

Nicki Minaj,
"Super Bass"

Coldplay,
"Every Teardrop
Is a Waterfall"

Adele,
"Someone
Like You"

Florence +
the Machine,
"Dog Days
Are Over"

Body Buffers: The proteins that keep you lean

Everyday Energizers: Sweet, tangy, high-energy fruit you should have at each meal

All-U-Can-Eat Anchors: Vegetables (have as much as you want!)

Crucial Carbs: Grains that whittle your waist

Herbs and Spices: Flavor enhancers (that satisfy without adding sugar, sodium, or major calories)

Each of these food categories has its own special properties that, when used together, create a foundation for continued, effective weight loss. I'll be detailing their benefits in the chapters ahead, but it's a very simple way to remember that if you fill your plate with these foods, you've done two things: You're making sure you're getting the right nutrients, and you're also pushing out all the bad that can easily creep into your diet.

Best of all, it works. One Harvard study tracked 120,000 people for two decades and found that the average adult gains about 3.5 pounds every four years. The ones who gained virtually no weight at all over that period? You got it. The ones who ate more fruits, vegetables, and whole grains—the very foods that make up a large part of your BEACH foods. Researchers speculate that foods that give you a satisfying balance of healthy fats, carbs, and protein, help keep you satiated, and thus, you're less likely to overeat. That, in a nutshell, is what the BEACH foods are all about: Satisfaction for both your taste buds and your belly.

SEXY STRATEGY #4:

Love Liquids

Take one look at the way we drink now and you've got a good snapshot of exactly what's wrong with the dietary habits that so many of us have today. It used to be simple: Coffee and juice in the morning, water or milk with meals, and perhaps a cocktail in the evening. Today? We've got more drink choices than crayon colors. Dozens of coffees, sodas, frapps, energy drinks, slushies, shakes, daiquiris, and more. Frankly, I'm surprised that some food manufacturer hasn't tried to sell a Thanksgiving dinner in a 16-ounce on-the-go drink. (Brilliant! That sound you hear now is a pack of food scientists scrambling back to the lab.)

Of course, this is for good reason: Drinks are easy (order and go). Drinks feel like they won't cost you anything calorically (so they feel healthy even if they're not). Drinks are part of (virtually) all things social. We not only have happy hour at night; we have it in the morning, too, except now it comes as a venti mocha calorie and sugar bomb.

Large Dairy Queen Oreo Blizzard

1,010 calories

YOU ATE IT? NEGATE IT!

110 minutes of swimming

The path down the beverage trail can be tricky. You can easily make drink choices that will blow your diet, especially if you make them every day. But I can also say that the right kinds of liquids can be part of the foundation of a good, waistline-friendly diet. What do I mean?

On this program, you will be embracing and enjoying soups and juices, because they can be packed with our BEACH foods, and as water-based liquids, they'll help fill you up so you feel satisfied (and can thus avoid being tempted by other cravings throughout the day). In one recent study, those who ate a soup-based meal experienced greater satiety than those who ate a mix of solids and liquids (the same meal, just one was turned into a soup). In the study, the emptying of the food from the digestive system was delayed, thus contributing to the greater feeling of fullness.

Now, by soups and juices, I don't mean pre-packaged ones, because canned or dehydrated soups are often loaded with sodium, and bottled juices are often just vehicles for extra sugar. On this plan, you'll be making nutritious and tasty soups and juices that will serve as meals. And with each spoonful or sip, you'll be shedding pounds even as you build better long-term health. A study review in the *International Journal of Food Sciences and Nutrition* found that pure fruit and vegetable

26

juices are associated with a reduced risk of both cancer and cardiovascular disease—health benefits that you'll experience as you embrace the Bikini Body Diet principles. A study published in the *European Journal of Nutrition* found that people who drank just one ounce of tart cherry juice a day reported that they slept longer and more soundly than those who didn't. And solid sleep isn't just good for your health. It's also great for your figure.

So your overall approach to liquids can be summed up in this way:

Maximize your intake of homemade juices and soups (rich in fruits and vegetables). A small Purdue University study published in the journal *Physiology & Behavior* found that soups provided the most satiety compared to liquids and solids with the same calorie content. The researchers explained that several factors can play a role—for one, soups generally have more macronutrients variety (a mix of protein and carbohydrates, for example) than most drinks and shakes typically do. And they also suggested that our brains play a role, too: We interpret soup as a meal, so our brains tell us that we're supposed to feel full after we eat them.

Drop soda, diet or not. According to a Gallup poll, 48 percent of Americans say they drink at least one soda every day. The non-diet ones, as you know, are nutritional disasters because of their high sugar content, and the diet ones also are linked to higher rates of obesity for a number of reasons. And a study from Denmark published in the *American Journal of Clinical Nutrition* looked at the storage of fat in people who drank regular soda, diet soda, low-fat milk, or water.

EMERGENCY CRAVING KILLER

Occassionally, you may be hit with the urge to eat something you shouldn't. Best to see if you can hold out (and plan it for your weekly cheat meal). Easier said than done. But if faced with that urge, take a walk or do a set of pushups. A study from the University of England found that people who took a 15-minute walk before sitting down to do a task while snacking ate half the amount of candy as those who took a break sitting at their desks. It's not only a distraction, but researchers say that the increased endorphins from physical activity can act as a stress-reliever and an appetite-killer.

Researchers found that after six months, the increase in fat storage (as well as total cholesterol) increased significantly in the two soda groups, even if they took in the same number of calories as the other groups.

A 2012 study published in the journal *Obesity* looked at the effects of both regular soda and diet soda on such things as waist size and fat percentage. Researchers found that regular soda was associated with increased waist size and abdominal fat, while diet soda was associated

What If I Cheat?

GOOD QUESTION. There are times when being unyieldingly strict can give you a sense of accomplishment and discipline. But sometimes, it can make you truly miserable, leaving you craving more of what you can't have. So sometimes, to save your sanity, it's OK to give yourself the green light to cheat—a little.

There also appears to be a benefit to having this kind of approach. The key to successful dieting is feeling as though you are in control of your food choices. New research from the *Journal of Consumer Research* shows that 80 percent of women who said, "I don't eat that," as opposed to, "I can't eat that," were able to resist foods not part of their plan. Only 10 percent of the "I can't" group was able to. The lesson: Knowing you're in control, rather than being mandated to follow everything to the letter, provides an important psychological benefit to make good choices throughout the day. So cheat, but only when you have made the conscious decision to do so. Absentmindedly plucking a creampuff off the passing dessert tray is not mindful cheating.

SO HERE ARE THE GUIDELINES FOR HOW FAR YOU SHOULD STRAY:

MEALS: After the 7-Day Super Slimdown during the first week, allow yourself one cheat meal per week after that. Plan it so that you know when it's coming (say, a holiday or a party or when you know you'll have a hard time sticking to your usual meals). If you plan it, you'll be more conscientious about what you can eat all week. It's best if your cheat meal is earlier in the day, but this isn't always realistic: I doubt you'll have chocolate truffles and champagne for breakfast.

That said, here's a fun fact for those who *do* want to make their cheat meal a breakfast: Researchers in Israel found that starting your day with a taste of dessert can help you lose weight. Those who added a treat to a well-balanced breakfast

with increased waist size, Body Mass Index (BMI), and total percentage of fat. And a study published in the journal *Diabetes Care* found that daily consumption of diet soda was associated with a 36 percent increased risk of metabolic syndrome and a 67 percent risk of developing type 2 diabetes. There are a number of theories why this may happen (after all, diet soda is zero calories, so how on earth could it be bad?). One of them: Because they have no calories, their sweet taste messes with our

lost 77 percent more weight than those who didn't have a splurge in the morning. Researchers suspect that because your metabolism is at its peak in the morning, you're better able to burn off those decadent foods throughout the day—and you might be less likely to crave them as the day progresses.

TREATS: Once a week, order a truly sinful dessert for your cheat meal. I mean an ice cream sundae extravaganza or a strawberry shortcake with nothing "short" about it. Make it your Friday night ritual. Cheating is part of life. (Just ask Don Draper.)

A great "sweet" and healthy way to satisfy your cravings is to invest in one of those fancy gourmet dark chocolate bars widely available today. Dark chocolate has many benefits, including helping to improve mood and also offering protection to your heart. The pros come from its plant source, the cacao bean, which contains flavanols (phytochemicals that act as antioxidants). But don't be fooled: Some products are labeled "dark chocolate" but have little if any

of the healthy nutrients left in them. Look for chocolate bars with at least 70 percent cacao. A new study published in the *Archives of Internal Medicine* found that those who ate cacao-based treats weighed less than those who at them infrequently. It may provide a metabolic boost. That said, the rest of the week, you need to keep your sweet tooth under tight control.

ALCOHOL: It's OK to have a daily glass of wine or clear liquor (except the first week). I'd suggest you even have the glass of wine at the end of your meal to help curb sweet cravings, if you have them. But you need to be careful: Several studies show that alcohol can increase appetite and food intake. One 2013 study review from Denmark published in the journal *Nutrition Reviews* suggests that intake of beer is associated with abdominal obesity, while a German study looking at nearly 160,000 women found that lifetime consumption of alcohol is positively related to abdominal fat.

hormonal systems, and our bodies crave sugar even more than if we had regular soda because our need for sugar hasn't been satisfied.

Make water or unsweetened green tea your standard drink with meals (sweeten with slices of fruit, if you like). According to a review of studies in the journal *PLoS One*, those who drank four or more cups of green tea a day were 16 percent less likely to be diagnosed with type 2 diabetes than nondrinkers. And a study in the *Journal of Nutrition* reported that people who drank green tea and exercised regularly burned more calories than those who exercised but didn't have the tea.

MY WORKOUT PLAYLIST

Ali Sweeney

AC/DC,
"Moneytalks"

Maroon 5,
"Harder to Breathe"

Fun.,
"Some Nights"

Foo Fighters,
"These Days"

All American Rejects,
"Gives You Hell"

(Just be careful of bottled tea; some can have as much added sugar as a Coke.) And when in doubt, drink water. A study in the journal *Obesity* found that increases in drinking water were associated with weight loss and fat loss. And a different study in the same journal found that simply replacing sweetened caloric drinks with water led to an average intake reduction of 200 calories a day. That equates to nearly a pound lost in two weeks from making just one swap.

Coffee is also fine, but minimize the additions. If you can drink it black, that's best. If not, try a little almond milk. Bonus: Caffeine can help boost your athletic performance in addition to your energy levels, according to a small British study. In that study, people who had about 180 milligrams of caffeine before working out did more reps of each exercise than those who didn't. (More on coffee on page 79.)

No booze during the 7-Day Super Slimdown, but an occasional drink after that is acceptable. In moderation, wine is fine, as are clear liquors like vodka. But no sugary mixers, like those used for daiquiris and margaritas. As you think about your own diet, consider this scary stat: People who consume alcohol get a crazy 16 percent of their daily calories from beer, wine, and other sources of booze. There's a big calorie-savings waiting if you fall into this category and can cut back to an average of one or fewer glasses a day. Though alcohol has been shown to have some benefits: In fact, a 2010 study published in the *Archives of Internal Medicine* found that normal-weight women who consumed a light or moderate amount of alcohol gained less weight and had a lower risk of becoming overweight or obese during nearly 13 years of follow-up than even non-drinkers. And a Harvard University study showed that women who drank five to seven drinks a week are 20 percent more likely to be free of major diseases and ailments late in life. The reasoning, according to the study authors: Alcohol in moderate amounts can improve cholesterol and reduce inflammation, and that can lower the risk of some diseases.

SEXY STRATEGY #5:

Reach for Reinforcements

We live in a world designed to help us undo our own mistakes. That's why we have spell-check, password retrieval systems, and "Are you sure you want to delete?" prompts. The reinforcements, though they sometimes complicate our lives (wrong again, smartphone autocorrect!), help protect us when we're vulnerable.

In your diet, then, it also makes sense to have backups—a support system—that can help in your quest toward achieving your healthy body goals. So here are some of the supplemental allies that will enhance the effects of the Bikini Body Diet:

Magnesium: This muscle relaxer helps you keep calm and promotes peaceful sleep. (As you'll see, sleep and energy are huge parts of making any diet plan work, so please don't minimize the importance of those elements in your life.) According to the National Institutes of Health, magnesium is needed for more than 300 chemical reactions in the body, including keeping the heart rhythm steady, regulating blood sugar levels, and helping lower blood pressure. A deficiency in magnesium has also been shown to have a direct relationship with some heart conditions, and some research suggests that a higher magnesium intake can reduce the risk of colon cancer. A 2013 study in the journal *Circulation* showed that low levels of magnesium were associated with the development of atrial fibrillation in people without cardiovascular disease. And many studies have shown that magnesium may help treat such conditions as osteoporosis, PMS, migraines, depression, and more.

1 serving of chocolate mousse
455 calories

YOU ATE IT?
NEGATE IT!

60 minutes of ballroom dancing

Besides those health benefits, magnesium can also aid in weight loss and body shaping. A 2013 study in the *Journal of Nutrition* found that higher magnesium intake was associated with lower levels of fasting glucose and insulin (markers related to fat and weight gain), and one study from England found that a magnesium supplement may have some beneficial effects on reducing fluid retention during the menstrual cycle, suggesting that it might help alleviate undesirable tummy bloat.

The recommend amount of magnesium for women under 30 is 310 milligrams, and 320 for women over 30. You'll find magnesium in many foods, including leafy green vegetables, beans, and nuts. Supplements in pill or powder form are also widely available at health food stores. I drink warm water with a tablespoon of magnesium powder every night before bed. It helps me sleep soundly and stay regular, reducing bloat and discomfort.

Vitamin D: Vitamin D has many benefits, yet most of us are deficient in it. (In fact, if you live north of Atlanta or Phoenix, studies show you're almost certain to be D-deficient most of the year.) I personally just had blood work done and learned I was severely D-deficient. So I take a vitamin D pill daily to supplement my diet. Why is this key? Studies suggest that vitamin D aids in increasing muscle strength, while having low levels of it is linked to such things as heart disease and cancer. Some research shows that people with low levels of vitamin D catch more colds or the flu than those with the highest amounts. That's a benefit itself, but think about the trickle effect, too: The more you get sick, the less you feel like exercising and the more susceptible you are to reaching for so-called feel-good foods.

But in terms of weight loss specifically, vitamin D may also play a promising role. Vitamin D helps regulate hunger and appetite. A 2012 Iranian study in *Nutrition Journal* found that supplementation with vitamin D was associated with a 7 percent decrease in fat, and a small study from the University of Minnesota found a relationship between higher levels of D and fat loss, especially in the belly area. Of course, that doesn't mean that taking vitamin D is a one-pill-cures-all. But to supplement your good exercise and eating habits, make sure you get the recommended amount every day through diet, sunlight (get at least 15 minutes outdoors, especially during winter months), and supplementation if necessary. You can get vitamin D in a variety of foods, such as fish, eggs, and fortified dairy products; the daily recommended intake is 600 IU. Research from the Cleveland Clinic shows you'll get better absorption of a vitamin D supplement if you take it with your largest meal.

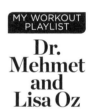

MY WORKOUT PLAYLIST

Dr. Mehmet and Lisa Oz

Foster the People,
"Pumped Up Kicks"

Alexandra Stan,
"Mr. Saxobeat"

Black Eyed Peas,
"I Gotta Feeling"

Fabolous,
"You Be Killin' 'Em"

Wiz Khalifa,
"Black and Yellow"

Bilberry and Probiotics: There are a million different supplements out there. Some folks believe they're magic bullets; others think the local vitamin store is nothing but a sham. But from my many years of studying supplements and their effects on the female body, there are two more that stand out as having true potential. Bilberry (related to the blueberry), for example, may provide beneficial effects due to its antioxidant properties. One 2011 study from the journal *Diabeteologia* found that a diet high in bilberry (as well as fatty fish and whole grains) improved function of the circulatory system (including improved blood pressure and other circulatory issues that are associated with being overweight).

Mounting research is drawing a connection between gut-health aids like probiotics—the healthy bacteria that live in our intestines or gut—and weight control. The ingestion of probiotics, either from foods like yogurt or supplements, has been shown to be effective at everything from boosting the immune system and reducing gastrointestinal problems to treating cancer. Research from the Washington University School of Medicine has linked obesity to a lack of gut flora diversity. Look for probiotic supplements with at least 5 billion active cells.

SEXY STRATEGY #6:

Target, Tone, and Torch

There's a reason why five of six principles of the Bikini Body Diet revolve around food: That's where weight-loss plans are won and lost. Have a strong nutritional approach and you'll develop a strong body. Have a weak one? And you could sweat like a Florida moving-company man but not make progress. Your diet is crucial to helping you lose fat.

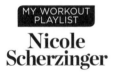

MY WORKOUT PLAYLIST

Nicole Scherzinger

Beyoncé,
"Run the World"

Adele,
"Rolling in the Deep"

Pitbull,
"Give Me Everything"

Michael Jackson,
"Dirty Diana"

Sly and the Family Stone,
"Everyday People"

Of course, you can accelerate that process, and also tone your body, by adding exercise into the mix.

Though women are often stereotyped as being the cardio-only gender, the fact is that you will be more successful at changing your body by doing both higher-intensity cardio work and some kind of strength training. That's why the Bikini Body Diet workout plan utilizes both. You will find details (and so many wonderfully effective routines) in upcoming chapters, but what we've found over and over again—through research, anecdotal success stories, and by prying into the workout routines of some of the world's most famously fit women—is that the combination of cardio and strength training allows your body to torch fat and tone trouble zones more effectively than one method alone. The workout plans in this book focus on those special bikini areas—your legs, butt, and core—that help give you a strong and sleek body. Best of all, they won't take a lot of your time, so you have no excuses to skip them.

I've spent the last decade studying exercise and its effect on a woman's body, and I've learned that there's one singular, most effective workout in the world: the one you're willing to stick with. So if you are addicted to your local group cycling or yoga class, and you're pleased with the results, don't change.

2 Fun-Size packs of M&M's
180 calories

But do consider supplementing what you already do with the workouts in this book. If you want the scientific answer to the question of the world's most effective workout, try this: It's one in which you raise your heart rate with interval training while also taxing your muscles with resistance training.

YOU ATE IT?
NEGATE IT!
60 minutes of yoga

For those who don't know, high-intensity interval training (HIIT) is a kind of cardiovascular exercise that alternates periods of high intensity and low intensity—sort of the workout equivalent of hot-water/cold-water baths at a spa. You can create a HIIT program with any type of exercise or equipment, be it running, swimming, cycling, rowing, or other forms of cardiovascular training. There are a number of ways to do this, and I'll outline them starting on page 132, but the point is that it's a little different than steady-state cardiovascular exercise, because you're really pushing your intensity and then throttling back, rather than going at one rate for an extended period of time. Quick note: There's absolutely nothing wrong with steady-state cardiovascular exercise, and I encourage you to do that, too, but much of the weight-loss research really centers around using these high-intensity activities as the best path for burning calories.

One study from the United Kingdom, published in the journal *Metabolism,* found that sprint training helped study participants lose inches from their waist and hips after just two weeks on the program, while a 2012 Italian study published in the *Journal of Translational Medicine* found that high-intensity interval training led to more calories burned post-exercise than traditional resistance training alone.

The Bikini Body Diet

And a University of Arkansas study found that those people who exercised with high intensity experienced a 20 percent decrease in abdominal fat, while those who exercised at a more traditional steady-state pace did not have any decrease.

By adding in resistance training, you'll double-up on both your calorie burn and your ability to gain some muscle (not bodybuilder muscle, but muscle that makes you toned and also uses energy to burn body fat). One University of Maryland study showed that your metabolic rate increases after weight training—so while you may not feel like you've sweated and huffed and puffed during a traditional weights workout, you're still getting the effects of amping up your metabolism.

With the Bikini Body Diet workouts, you will work your tushy off (quite literally), in a short but intense amount of time. One of the challenges in any weight-loss plan is not just having the physical energy to train, but also squeezing in sessions. That's another reason why these high-intensity and strength workouts work so well—you can get the most bang for your (workout) buck.

And while only you can determine the best exercise schedule for your own life, if you want an extra nudge, work out first thing in the morning: Researchers at Brigham Young University found that those who worked out earlier in the day showed less brain activity when exposed to photos of food later, compared to those who didn't exercise before seeing the same photos. While researchers are unclear of why that happened, they said that exercising can alter hunger-controlling hormones. So working out early may give you a bit of an advantage in managing those cravings as the day goes on.

BRING ON THE BIKINI BODY!

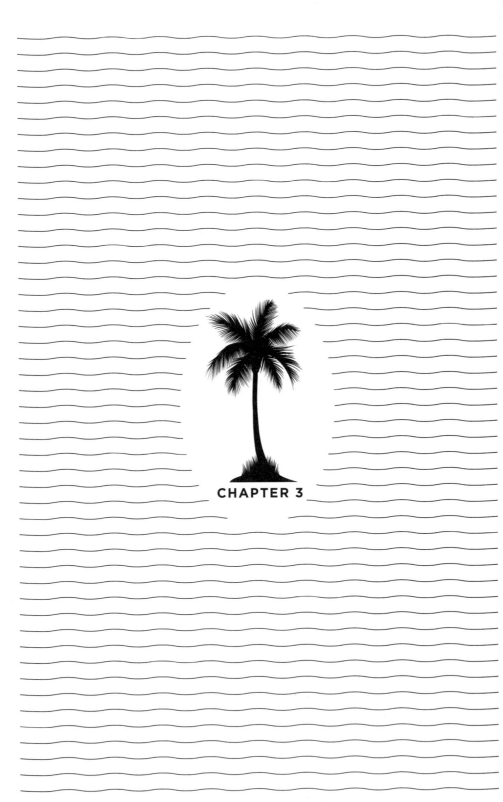

CHAPTER 3

A Bikini Body Is a Healthy Body!

How Improving Your Looks Will Improve Your Life

There's no doubt that you may read the title of this book and think that it's just about looking good. Heck, that's what bikinis are all about, right? Cover up little, show off lots! (Few things are more revealing than a bikini.) So yes, of course, I admit it: There's a huge "looking good" factor to this diet and plan. Let's be frank: Who really hits the gym a 6:30 a.m. simply for an endorphin rush? It's to fit into those skinny jeans and make your skin glow.

39

The Bikini Body Diet

But here's what's really working underneath, and what you should care about just as much as the mirror: The Bikini Body Diet is about your heart, your muscles, your blood vessels, your internal organs, your cells, and your brain, too. It's about your health.

Now, internal organs and bikinis may seem like they go together about as well as plaid and polka dots, but they do. This diet is about embracing eating and exercise patterns that strengthen you inside and out. The eating and exercise plans, in fact, employ foods and activities that will not only change your looks, but also how your entire body works, so that you can live longer and healthier. So yes, while I do want you, over the course of these six weeks, to feel better about your changing bod, I also want you to embrace the fact that these changes are doing more than helping you drop inches and pounds.

They're also helping add years to your life—and happy ones at that!

You already know some of the scary facts: About 45 million Americans start a diet every year. Yet, by the year 2030, if trends continue, 42 percent of Americans will be obese. That's a scary statistic, so something clearly is not working. We have more and more people trying to diet, and more and more people failing. We all know that the blame falls into a number of categories: A combination of bad eating habits, sedentary behavior, aging (hello, slowed metabolism), and complex psychological and emotional factors that contribute to our weight, size, and shape problems.

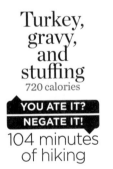

Turkey, gravy, and stuffing
720 calories

YOU ATE IT?
NEGATE IT!

104 minutes of hiking

But what makes these facts truly worrisome isn't the fact that our beaches and pools (and, yes, mirror reflections) are getting less visually appealing. What we really need to worry about are the health consequences of this growing problem, from diabetes and high blood pressure to cardiovascular disease and cancer. (Women with higher body fat have increased estrogen, which can contribute to tumor growth.)

Also, abdominal obesity is riskier than if you carry your weight in your butt or thighs. Research shows that the fat nearest to your organs (in the form of extra abdominal fat) puts you at increased risk of hypertension, diabetes, and cardiovascular disease. One of the reasons: Because that belly fat is so close to your internal organs, it simply pumps them full of toxins. And here's a scary stat: Researchers from the University of Oxford found that excess fat can enter your bloodstream and be stored by the cells around your waistline in as little as three hours. (It is, however, the kind of tissue that can be burned off, but over time, the excess stakes a permanent place on your belly.)

MY WORKOUT PLAYLIST

Mariska Hargitay

The Rolling Stones, "Start Me Up"

Jason Mraz, "I'm Yours"

Jay-Z featuring Alicia Keys, "Empire State of Mind"

Michael Jackson, "Thriller

Sheryl Crow, "Out of Our Heads"

Another fact: If your waist size is more than half your height in inches, your projected lifespan is shorter than those whose waistlines are not, according to obesity research.

What we have to do is shift our thinking so that while we acknowledge the problem, we focus on what the solution will bring. By following the Bikini Body Diet principles, you will not only see nearly immediate sleekifying benefits, but you will also see a change in your overall health. In fact, it's why targeting the trouble zones—especially your belly—is a critical part of this plan.

Consider some of these important facts: Even a 5- to 10-pound weight loss will help you start seeing health benefits, with drops in blood pressure, cholesterol, blood sugar—and ultimately risk of other diseases, too. According to a study published in the *Journal of the American Medical Association*, if you exercise for two and a half hours every week, you could be 13 pounds skinnier than someone who doesn't work out. The more intense and more frequent, the better. And a review published in the *International Journal of Clinical Practice* found that regular exercise can prevent more than 25 diseases and health conditions down the road. For example, workouts lower the risk of:

➤ Breast cancer by 30 percent

➤ Colon cancer by 40 percent

➤ Depression by 28 percent

➤ Heart disease by 50 percent

➤ Hip fractures by 41 percent

Those numbers—not 36-24-36—are the ones that really matter.

When you think of the big diseases that change lives (and end them), you can see what role fat plays. Consider blood pressure, for example. As you know, blood pressure is all about having good blood flow throughout your body, as your heart pumps blood and circulates it up and down and all around—to help fuel your body and make sure all organs and systems run smoothly. But let's say you've had one too many pieces of chocolate cake. (And by "one," I mean "many.") You start to build up plaque in your arteries, which acts as a roadblock to blood flow. Arteries and veins begin to stiffen. Blood can't flow as freely, so the pressure rises and rises, which means your heart has to pump harder and harder, causing stress and strain on your ticker. That's what leads to heart attack, heart failure, and stroke. "Chocolate cake" no longer sounds so great, right?

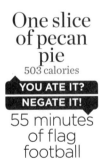

One slice
of pecan
pie
503 calories

YOU ATE IT?
NEGATE IT!

55 minutes
of flag
football

A similar biological process happens when it comes to diabetes (type 2 adult-onset), which has a major association with obesity. In this case, when you consume too many calories, your body gets bombarded with blood sugar (glucose). Your body tries to handle it via insulin, the hormone that helps transport the glucose from your bloodstream for use throughout your body as energy. As you overeat, your system is flooded again and again with insulin, until your cells eventually come to feel about this critical hormone the way you came to feel about your ex with a wandering eye— you develop a resistance. When your cells no longer respond eagerly to insulin, you can't process glucose properly and remove it from your bloodstream—and glucose is toxic to your circulatory system.

So I don't think there's any question about what's at stake here:

Ultimately, bikini bodies are healthy bodies. And there's no greater confidence-booster than knowing your sexiness goes hand-in-hand with being strong and healthy.

However, one of the central questions many women have is, "How do I get there?"

Look on the Bright Side, and Get Your Body on the Light Side

In a survey of 1,000 people, 9 out of 10 who thought positively about the health benefits of dieting lost or maintained their weight over a year. Those who took a more negative approach toward dieting? Only 5 of 10 participants lost or maintained weight.

That's very revealing—and shows the strong ties between mind and body. If you can go into a diet and exercise plan with a positive approach (and an understanding that you will face obstacles), you will have a much higher chance of maintaining it than if you focus on the downs or the mini-setbacks that you experience.

While everyone has different personalities and approaches and responds to diets in different ways, many women can steer their attitudes in the right direction with one simple change: Grab a partner. Too many of us try to go it alone. But something magical happens when you take a team approach to dieting and exercise. It's different. It feels good. You want to succeed. You want to lean on someone and be there for her, too. Now, I know I can't automatically tap you on the shoulder and ask you to be all sunny and happy and say, "Hey, bikini shopping tomorrow!" But I can encourage you to stop the thinking that dieting has to be secret or private or something to be ashamed of.

I know that this played a huge role for me as I prepared for my photo shoot. Knowing that I had the support of the staff around me, who I could talk to and even lean on, helped me tremendously to get through the times when I just wanted to curl up and say, forget it, it's just easier to down the whole pint of rocky road right here and right now.

Plus, the support doesn't have to be overt. It doesn't have to come in the form of constant phone calls or drill-sergeant tactics telling you to get your butt moving and do another 500 burpees right this instant. Just knowing you do have people—and aren't hiding your plan and goal—is often all you need to make that mental switch from "Woe is me" to "Let's do this."

Focus on the goals; focus on the changes happening on the inside of your body even if they're not always happening quickly on the outside. Focus on the fact that you are working toward your goal. Keep those thoughts at the front of your mind to push out the discouraging ones. That foundation will help you stay on the right path.

I can't tell you how to think or how to feel, but a positive belief system is a fundamental part of having success on any weight-loss or body-changing program. Is it easy to do? Not always. A few simple acts of healthy living and a few days during which you change your approach to exercise and eating can be enough to kick-start not only your body, but your brain as well—hence the 7-Day Super Slimdown.

Sleep Away Pounds

When it comes to changing your diet, one of the hardest things to change might not even be your eating habits—like opting for grilled chicken rather than a greasy burger—but may be getting enough sleep.

It's a fact: Women don't sleep enough, and it's killing our bodies. And not just in the mentally exhausted "I'm tired all day" kind of way; but in the physically tangible, visible "My jeans won't button" kind of way.

Yes, there are times when we just can't get enough sleep. In our busy, plugged-in world, it's hard to shut off and shut down. There's more to do—

always. At work, at home, on Facebook. We'd rather live than slumber. That is, until morning comes, the alarm sounds, and oh, how we wish we could sleep for just...a...few...more...minutes. But we can't. So we get up, try to pep ourselves up with a 32-ounce milkshake disguised as "coffee," and think we'll be better, until the afternoon comes and we nearly fall asleep on our keyboards. So we order up some more of our favorite caffeine-

HIDDEN CAUSES OF WEIGHT GAIN

Many women know why they've gained weight. In short, it usually comes down to too much food and not enough exercise. But that's not always the case. There can be other root causes of weight gain. If you feel as if your eating and exercise is typically in good shape but you're not, you may want to do some further investigating to see whether there are other biological forces at work. Some of the most common (yet often secret) ones for women:

CONDITION	WHAT HAPPENS	OTHER SYMPTONS	TREATMENT
Polycystic Ovarian Syndrome (PCOS)	Hormonal imbalances lead to overload of insulin, which increases fat storage	Unusually light, heavy, or missing periods; breakouts; facial hair; abdominal fat	Medication called Metformin can control insulin levels. Eat smaller meals every few hours to move sugar into muscles without insulin.
Underactive Thyroid	If the thyroid gland doesn't produce enough hormones that control metabolism, body burns fat sluggishly	Feeling of being tired and cold, constipation, puffiness in legs and face	Doc will likely prescribe a synthetic version of T3 and T4 hormones
Stress	The body releases the hormone cortisol, which triggers you to store calories as fat in preparation for hard times	Sleep trouble, high blood pressure, headaches	Take five deep, controlled breaths to keep cortisol from spiking
Medication Side Effects	Some prescription meds can stimulate appetite	Antidepressants and steroids are often associated with weight gain	Ask your doc about switching meds; there are many on the market that work in a similar fashion

infused treat and carry on. And, oh, while we're at it, that 7,000-calorie bagel sandwich looks pretty good, too.

And the cycle repeats itself over and over. Fewer hours of sleep means more food calories. Simple. Consider this: According to a study in the *American Journal of Epidemiology*, women who slept five hours or fewer per night were 32 percent more likely to experience major weight gain over 16 years than those who got more sleep. Why? Too little sleep causes an increase in a hormone that stimulates appetite (that's called ghrelin). And according to a study from the New York Obesity Nutrition Research Center, when women got four hours of sleep instead of eight, they consumed more than 300 extra calories a day—mostly from fatty foods. A study from the Mayo Clinic in Minnesota found that an 80-minute shortcoming in sleep can lead to people eating on average 550 more calories the next day.

Peanut-butter sandwich crackers
220 calories per 6-pack
YOU ATE IT? NEGATE IT!
76 minutes of hatha yoga

So while you may be making some changes to your diet and exercise habits, ask yourself whether you're getting enough quality sleep. And if the answer is no, then do an assessment of your sleeping and lifestyle patterns to identify what the problems may be, such as too much caffeine or working too closely to bedtime. Making this change alone will do wonders for your weight-loss goals. Getting enough quality sleep will help stop the domino effect that happens when you don't. Instead of seeking sugar-laden foods, your body will be primed for the day with innate energy.

Sometimes, we sacrifice sleep and think we can out-muscle our bodies to hang on and get our work done, but it's absolutely one of the worst things we can do—not just for our energy, but for our waistlines, as well. There's a direct correlation between decreased sleep hours and increased clothes sizes. When we can't sleep or nap, we're forced to find other ways to power through the day. So we eat.

There are a number of strategies you can use to fall asleep easier so you get those seven to eight hours. Try these:

Ditch all electronics in the bedroom. Screen time is both stimulating and it emits a blue hue that mimics daylight, which is not good when trying to fall asleep. Go gadget-less an hour before bed to start your wind-down.

Keep the bedroom cool. Your body sleeps best in temps around 65 degrees, give or take a few degrees. It's the temperature at which your body can stay in a normal state without having to shiver or perspire.

Take a look at some of your habits throughout the day. Maybe you need to ditch caffeine if you have it in the afternoon (it can stay in your system for up to 12 hours). Or maybe you should exercise in the morning or at lunch if you're an evening exerciser. A recent study presented to the American College of Sports Medicine found that 7 a.m. workouts improved sleep quality more than late-day sessions did.

Take a shower. Heating your skin and then stepping into a cool room can serve as a body signal that it's time for sleep.

Fight it. Instead of telling yourself "I need to fall asleep, I need to fall asleep, I need to fall asleep," turn the argument on its head. Grab a book and tell yourself you need to stay awake for another 30 minutes. You may soon find yourself dozing off. Reverse psychology works on yourself, too!

Get up around the same time every day—even on the weekend. If you throw your schedule too far off during the weekends, your body can't get into a regular routine, and it'll throw off your snoozing patterns for the whole week.

Sniff some lavender, which has been shown to improve sleep quality, according to a Wesleyan University study. Researchers found that people who took a whiff of lavender oil before bed awoke with more energy (and spent more time in deep sleep) than those who didn't. Some other tactics: A glass of warm milk (because it contains some amounts of sleep-friendly tryptophan), or a glass of tart cherry juice, which contains the sleep hormone melatonin. A British study found that those who drank it regularly slept longer and more deeply than those who didn't.

Not only will better sleep help improve your health, but if you aren't getting good sleep, any diet plan will feel like swimming upstream. You'll be fighting biological forces that make it virtually impossible to fuel your body with the nutrients that will get you through the day and help power your workouts.

It's All About Renewable Energy

Both of these issues—a healthy attitude and high-quality sleep—really boil down to one issue, the one that's critical whenever you're striving to change your body: Energy.

The nutrition and exercise plans I outline in this book are designed to flood your body with the energy and power to succeed. Without that energy, it will be tough; that's why a positive attitude and a healthy amount of sleep are so important to your quest.

Another way to think about it: Consider all the sources of energy you use around the house and at work every day. Electrical power, battery power, gas power, and all other forms, too. Each one is important. And our individual bodies are a little like that, too. We garner most of our energy from food—the higher quality the foods, the better the energy source. But we also garner it from other places, too, like exercise and having enough sleep. And when one of your energy systems fails, falters, or isn't up to the task of keeping you going, it affects your other energy systems.

So what happens if you flip the negative energy cycle? Where good energy leads to more energy, which leads to better decisions, which leads to a good attitude, which leads to excitement, which leads to more energy, and so on, and so on, and so on?

What if your energy level and positive attitude about the changes you're making build on one another, rather than allowing mini-setbacks to become majors ones?

The answer to those "what if" questions are waiting for you in a dressing room near you.

May I suggest a pretty pink one to start?

CHAPTER 4

Your Brain
and
Belly
Fat

"Lean and Healthy" Is a State of Mind— Literally

Here's a question with an easy answer:

What are the two major components of a diet plan? Food and exercise, right?

Cut back on the bad foods, increase the good ones, and work your booty off. That's the formula for success.

And, yes, if we wanted to boil diets down to those major factors, we'd all be right. But what often gets lost in the talk of protein and pushups is that

51

weight-management is not only about the belly or the heart or the rectus abdominis. It's about what's happening in the brain. The mental part. All those things that influence what we think and feel about food, whether we choose to exercise or crawl back into bed, how we decide to attack each and every day. Yes, it's about the food. Yes, it's about the exercise. But it's also about whether you're in the state of mind to make changes to your life—ones that make changes to your body possible.

Emotions are everything. They influence our behavior all day, every day. And the negative ones can be dangerous.

Sometimes, we don't talk about them. Sometimes, we don't even know we have them. But the mind plays a role in how and what we eat (ice cream being one of life's most popular soothers and all...).

When it comes to stress and depression, we often think that we should just be able to will ourselves out of a funk. But the truth is that there are real chemical processes taking place that affect the way our bodies reacts to temptation. And that makes sense, right? How you feel certainly influences whether you're motivated to eat well or would rather throw in the towel and order a croque madame.

As part of our holistic system of appetite and energy, our hormones are essentially communicating with each other: Don't feel so well? Yes, let's eat. Under a pile of work with belligerent bosses on your back? One hand's on the keyboard, the other in a bag of chocolate-covered pretzels. And it's not something that you can just will yourself beyond; these are biological reactions inside your body that trigger your actions.

Manage Your Stress, Manage Your Waist

Too often, we like to package stress as something we can completely eliminate. If only we didn't have problems, we'd be thin. If only we didn't have to be pulled in different directions. If only we could live on a tropical island, then we'd have a bikini body. It's a nice idea, isn't it? But

it's not a realistic one. We all have stress, and it can come in all forms—
be it with your family, your work, your umbrella breaking at the absolute worst time. But guess what? As humans, we're equipped to handle

HIDDEN SIGNS OF STRESS

Most of the time, we know when we're stressed. After all, is it that hard to
know that we're behind deadline or late to Junior's soccer practice when
everybody and their mother is buzzing and beeping and texting and tweeting
that we are? Sometimes, though, stress manifests itself not just in that
"Backoff, world" feeling you may get. It also comes in the form of pain
and tension throughout your body. Here's the lowdown:

THE PAIN	WHAT'S HAPPENING	WHAT TO DO FOR RELIEF
Jaw	Pain radiating from the side of the face to the head or neck can be TMJ (temporomandibular joint disorder). Many times, it's caused by clenching your teeth while under stress.	Open your jaw wide, hold, then let it relax. Try to make it a habit to hold your jaw open slightly so your teeth don't touch.
Lower Back	It can be caused by everything from poor posture to long hours of sitting, but some research shows that women who report signs of stress are more likely to experience back pain.	Stand with your heels and shoulders touching a wall. Tilt your pelvis back, so the small of the back presses against the wall, relieving back muscles. Hold for 15–30 seconds. Do this regularly to ease some tension. Also strengthening your abdominal muscles will help support your back muscles.
Neck	A lot of us hold tension in our necks, often causing pain to radiate to the shoulders.	While sitting in a chair, lower your chin to your chest, letting the weight of your head gently stretch the tense muscles. Rotate your head to each side.
Headaches	Tension headaches occur all around the head, though it's most intense at the temples and back of the skull.	Try a self-massage technique: Gently press fingers on both sides of face around the hinge of jaw, rubbing in a circular motion. Next, move hands to the area just behind the jaw and below the ears, and gently slide hands down your neck to the base of your shoulders. Repeat.

stress. That's how we get our work done, that's how we cope, that's one of the things that makes us human—our intellectual and creative ability to solve all of life's complex problems.

The bigger picture, though, is that we're not equipped to handle long-term stress—that is, stress that keeps pounding and pounding and pounding us, like waves on a rocky coastline. When we're under chronic stress, that's when our hormonal systems go bonkers and we seek to quiet the storm with a pint of caramel syrup.

Chemically, here's what happens: When we're stressed, our body releases high levels of the stress hormone cortisol, which causes a cascade of chemical processes that ultimately lead us to search for energy (in the form of calories) that will calm us. Often those foods come in the form of simple and sugary carbohydrates as a way to boost levels of the feel-good hormone dopamine, which then has a cascading effect: Need more dopamine? Eat more doughnuts! Feel bad about doughnuts? Find more dopamine! Drink a martini. And so on...

1 large movie popcorn
1,200 calories
YOU ATE IT? NEGATE IT!
87 minutes of group cycling

But the issue of stress doesn't just have to do with your wanting to call up the pizza man, gorge on three slices, and then call him back and berate him for bringing it in the first place. It has to do with the chemical and hormonal reactions that can happen in your body that cause you to store fat in your belly.

As cortisol increases (when stress increases), your body goes into a sort of panic mode: It thinks it's under duress and figures it needs to hold onto some of its energy (in case it needs to use that energy if none is available, as would be in the case of a famine). What's the easiest way for your body to do that? Store that fat close to your belly so that energy is at the ready. Only problem? We're not living in a society where you'll go days or weeks without food. You can completely replenish your calories and constantly fuel your body with energy sources. So that fat that got stored close to your belly in case of an emergency? Turns out, there's no emergency. Just more and more stress, more and more fat storage, and no need to use it. So it becomes the most vicious of cycles: Get stressed, eat. Eat too much, store fat. Stay stressed, eat more and store more, which actually triggers a cycle that causes you to store even more fat. Repeat and repeat and repeat...

That throws off lots of different chemical and hormonal systems in the body, making it increasingly difficult to lose fat in these tough spots. (Side note: For women entering menopause and seeing decreased estrogen levels, those declines also appear to contribute to fat storage in the belly area.)

Research supports this relationship between stress and weight gain. One study published in the *American Journal of Epidemiology* followed more than 1,300 people for nine years. Those who reported higher levels of stress showed increases in waist size and weight. And what's worse, it seems as though gaining weight under stress actually trains your body to gain weight even more efficiently: Those who had the highest Body Mass Index numbers (which measure the relationship between weight and height) reported the most weight gain when under increased stress. And surveys from the American Psychological Association show that nearly half of people admit to eating bad foods (or overeating) when faced with stressful situations.

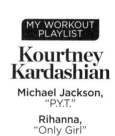

MY WORKOUT PLAYLIST

Kourtney Kardashian

Michael Jackson,
"P.Y.T."

Rihanna,
"Only Girl"

P!nk,
"So What"

The Beatles,
"Hey Jude"

Kanye West,
"All the Lights Out"

Stress, and all of its related mental and emotional issues, doesn't come with easy answers. Sometimes, the best way to "manage" stress is to fix the problem, whether it's a head-on confrontation about family tension or changing jobs or something else that can be a major moment in your life. After all, you can't solve all your stress with a bubble bath. That said, it is important for your body to know that you are trying to calm the storm. And even some simple stress-management techniques can have a strong impact on how your body handles anxiety (and, ultimately, how it handles storing fat).

SOME TACTICS FOR HELPING YOU DEAL WITH LIFE'S STRESSORS:

✳ Smiling is an instant stress-buster, according to a recent study in *Psychological Science.* You can use it anytime, anywhere.

✳ A recent study from the *Journal of Nutrition* found that dehydration contributes to stress and low energy levels, so it's important to stay hydrated with water (no calories!). Will this wash away your problems? Of course not, but maintaining energy levels is an essential aspect of dealing with the tasks of life and reaching your physical and emotional goals.

✳ As little as six minutes of reading can cut your feelings of stress by up to 60 percent, according to British researchers.

✳ People who took omega-3 supplements daily for 12 weeks reported their anxiety levels dropped by 20 percent, according to research from the Ohio State University.

✳ Find an activity that can allow you to do mini-meditations. Maybe it's a hike or walk. A new study published in *BMC Public Health* found that a 20-minute walk outside twice a week was more restorative than getting the same exercise indoors.

✳ The tried-and-true deep-breathing technique is a good one for a reason. It helps calm your nervous system. Take slow, deep breaths, counting one for inhale and one for exhale for a full minute.

✳ A University of Wisconsin-Madison study showed that hearing your mother's voice can lower levels of cortisol and trigger the release of the bonding hormone called oxytocin. But simply connecting with friends (especially if your mother's voice is the source of your stress!) can also do the trick and ease tension levels.

✹ Take 15-minute breaks every hour from your phone. A British study found that compulsively checking e-mails and texts can produce anxiety.

✹ Get your whole body in on the action with a deep stretch. A forward bend is perfect because it decompresses the spine and improves circulation, which helps release tension from your upper body (not to mention your mind). To do one, stand with your feet hip-width apart, then bend your knees slightly and fold your body forward. Grasp opposite elbows and let your head drop; hold for one minute. Another good way to release tension is to contract your muscles and then release them, because they're better able to fully relax after being under tension: Take a few deep breaths and then contract your right arm as tightly as you can, holding for two or three seconds. As you exhale, relax completely and let your arm drop. Repeat with other body parts and then your entire body.

✹ Another good reason to get enough sleep (in the form of a cat nap): A study in the *International Journal of Behavioral Medicine* found that adults who slept 45 minutes or more during the day had lower blood pressure and heart rate after completing a tough mental task than those who didn't get any shut-eye. If a nap is out of the question, try to add in that time at night

Improve Your Food, Improve Your Mood

Depression isn't like a broken bone: It's not as if you're either depressed or you're not. There's an entire spectrum of mood states. Some may be associated with hormonal cycles in women, and some are affected by everything from seasonal patterns to what's happening in your life on any given day. And we all know that having any form of depression—from mild to serious—influences everything we do. How we relate to people. How we work. How we eat. That's because the neurotransmitters that control mood, thinking, appetite, and behavior get all out of whack. And you seek comfort in the things that might make you feel good in the short term, even if they have damaging effects in the long term.

Depression can be hard to recognize and treat, but it is important to see your doctor if you have one or more of these symptoms for more than two weeks, because it could be a sign of severe depression.

* Persistent sad, anxious, or empty feelings
* Feelings of hopelessness or helplessness
* Guilty feelings
* Irritability, restlessness
* Fatigue, decreased energy
* Difficulty concentrating or performing other cognitive functions
* Insomnia, early waking, or excessive sleeping
* Overeating, appetite loss
* Thoughts of suicide
* Persistent aches or pains, headaches, cramps, or digestive problems that don't ease with treatment

Depression makes us eat poorly, skip exercising, and gain weight. Eating well and exercising help us lose weight and also fight depression. But you need a simple plan that will help you break the funk and take control of your life. And that's what the Bikini Body Diet is designed to do.

The Bikini Body Diet BEACH foods put you in control of your diet and your life, and just the practice of making smart choices can take your health—physical and mental—to a whole new level. Meanwhile, the Bikini Body Diet workout will help boost feel-good endorphins and energy, which will thus improve mood.

Another great mood-booster: Encourage a friend or family member to join you on your quest for a bikini body. Having a social support system improves levels of the feel-good hormone oxytocin. Essentially, what you're trying to do is find ways to satisfy that dopamine system I talked about earlier in relation to stress. So satisfaction may come in the form of a hobby, or a good conversation, or hanging with the family. What you're doing, essentially, is trying to shift that dopamine system so it can derive satisfaction from other things in your life, not nacho chips.

Milk chocolate
210 calories per 1.5-oz bar
YOU ATE IT? NEGATE IT!
28 minutes of hip-hop dancing

But that's not saying that food can't be of some help. In fact, there are plenty of Bikini Body Diet–friendly foods that have been shown to improve mood. Include more of these on your plate to keep those happy chemicals high and the hunger ones low.

Some options (which are also part of your BEACH foods):

Walnuts: We have long known that they're good for heart health, but new research shows that walnuts (along with almonds and hazelnuts) can also boost levels of serotonin, which helps put you in a good mood.

Chickpeas: They contain lots of folate, which is a type of B vitamin that is needed to produce dopamine—a neurotransmitter that's most often associated with pleasure.

Salmon, Tuna, and Sardines: Fatty, cold-water fish contains omega-3 fats, which can make you feel calmer. In one study, people who regularly ate foods high in omega-3s were 20 percent less anxious than those who didn't. And according to a study by the Ohio State University, for those people who took an omega-3 supplement for 12 weeks, anxiety levels dropped by 20 percent.

Avocados: They contain B vitamins, which help create that feel-good serotonin. Since stress depletes stores of B vitamins, avocados will help keep your tank full. They also have potassium (which helps lower blood pressure).

Sunflower Seeds: They have loads of magnesium, which is good because a magnesium deficiency can lower your dopamine (and this makes you feel more stressed and anxious).

Water: If you're dehydrated, you're more likely to feel more tired and stressed, and have less energy, according to a study from the *Journal of Nutrition*. And that can, of course, contribute to overeating.

Dark Chocolate: About 40 grams of dark chocolate (about four squares of a large bar) made from 75 percent cocoa reduced levels of stress hormones, according to a study published the *Journal of Proteome Research*.

Clearly, all is not going to be right with the world just because you popped a couple of pieces of dark chocolate and ordered salmon, so I'm not trying to imply that there are quick fixes to mood issues. But mood, like stress, is part of that energy system I talked about in the last chapter. When all of your systems are being fed with healthy forms of energy (in the form of BEACH foods), then they all work together to create a health body and mind.

Tell the World of Your Weight-Loss Quest

Many women first have to figure out the underlying sources of stress and depression and address them (and not assume they're going to just go down the drain along with the bath salts). That has to come first.

5 marsh-mallow Peeps
170 calories
YOU ATE IT? NEGATE IT!
21 minutes on rowing machine

One of the ways to do that is by taking your efforts public. Now, I'm not saying you have to take an ad out in the local paper or blog about your ups and downs for the world to read, though, for some, that can be fun, too. (People who used Twitter and Facebook as part of their weight-loss program were more successful than those who did not, according to some research.) And I'm not saying that you have to do what I did and agree to pose in a bikini for the whole world to see.

But what I am saying is that you should be sharing your story—and your journey—with at least one other person. If you want to keep it private, that's, of course, up to you. But after seeing hundreds and hundreds of success stories and talking to many celebrities about their weight-loss efforts, I know that there's a common thread: a sense of pride and accountability that comes into play when your body goals become even somewhat public. Remember, I don't define public as "millions." I define it as "at least one other person besides yourself."

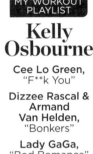

MY WORKOUT PLAYLIST

Kelly Osbourne

Cee Lo Green,
"F**k You"

Dizzee Rascal &
Armand
Van Helden,
"Bonkers"

Lady GaGa,
"Bad Romance"

Will.I.Am &
Nicki Minaj,
"Check It Out"

Girls Aloud,
"Sexy!
No No No..."

One of the reasons why so many diet program and weight-loss goals have failed is because they're missing that support system—those one, two, five, or 10 people who can relate to what you're going through or who want to go through it with you or who can just act as a sounding board when you feel guilty about "friending" both Ben and Jerry with a pint and a large spoon.

This "healthy-eating entourage," no matter how big or small, not only will help you with the larger issues in life, but it will also help keep you on track and be understanding if you have a few hiccups along the way. Much research shows that support systems simply work.

But too often, we go at it alone. So, yes, while I'll spend a lot of time talking about nutrients, butt muscles, flat tummies, and the reason why I love soups and juices so much, I also think that if the mind is right, the body will follow.

So this will then work twofold: By including others in your journey, you'll be building a support system that will help keep stress and depression at bay, but you'll also be using the very tool that may very well be the key to successfully following through on a weight-loss plan— the accountability that comes from involving other people. No, social interaction isn't labeled with a "Burns 40 calories an hour" sign or an "Only 3 grams of fat per serving" label. But the effect of other people on your quest may be exactly what you need. After all, baring it all in a bikini isn't just a matter of looking great—it's about self-esteem. And that's really at the heart of the Bikini Body Diet. We're all going to have different bikinis. We're all going to have different bodies. But we all share the same goal: Having the confidence to feel happy and proud of what we have.

CHAPTER 5

Your BEACH Foods

The 5 Bikini Body Diet Food Groups That Will Super-charge Your Path to Leanness

Remember the "Freshman 15"? It's the mysterious number on the scale that appears seemingly out of nowhere when a woman goes off to college for the first time (and the phenomenon is similarly common in women who go straight into the workforce after high school). Suddenly free of the structured eating system they grew up with, young women are faced with long nights, high stress, delivery pizza, keg parties, and rows of cafeteria machines dispensing streams of sugar- and calorie-laden desserts.

Funny thing is (actually, it's not so funny), we always talk about the Freshman 15, but we never talk about the Twenties 20, the Thirties 30, or the Forties 40. Our lives—as we get older, as we get busier, as our metabolisms slow down—enter a seemingly inexorable march toward gaining weight. But that march doesn't have to be your fate. If you re-learn how to eat, you can combat all the forces conspiring to make you fat.

It all starts—and ends—with BEACH foods. Follow the six major eating and exercise principles, and center your meals around the BEACH foods, and you'll be doing exactly what you should be doing to have the healthiest body possible. I developed the BEACH foods way of thinking because, one, it's an easy-to-remember device that will help guide all of your food choices; and two, it's a reminder about what you're after: a body built for baring at the beach.

What follows is a description of each category with some of the possible choices that fall under them (don't worry, you're not expected to remember them all). As long as you understand the major categories, you'll learn to navigate the tricky areas of supermarkets and restaurants alike. This is the way I eat, and I love it. So many flavors, so many choices. And in the next chapter, you'll see how they all work together in our delicious recipes.

Body Buffers—Muscle-building proteins

Everyday Energizers—Fruits (eat a serving at each meal)

All-U-Can-Eat Anchors—Vegetables (as much as you want)

Crucial Carbs—Good grains (there are healthy ones)

Herbs and Spices—Flavor enhancers without the calories

Pretty simple, right? But in fact, the BEACH foods are built on a scientific (and real-women-tested) series of principles that help create the optimal weight-loss nutrition zone day in and day out.

Before we get into the specifics, it's important to take a quick look at the science of how food travels through our digestive system, how it's used, and how it turns to fat. While most people just want to know the "what" to eat, understanding a little of the "why" and "how" helps you think about the process of eating.

Food, as you know, is energy. Your body needs that food not just to make you feel full of energy, but also to power all the systems and organs in your body. We get that energy in three major forms—protein, fat, and carbohydrates, also known as the macronutrients. While some people like to simplify the process (fat turns into fat and protein only builds muscle), it's not quite that cut-and-dried. In fact, any food can be stored as fat if it's not used up by the body when it's digested. And most foods are, in reality, some combination of two or three of those macronutrients.

6-piece chocolate sampler
408 calories

YOU ATE IT? NEGATE IT!
35 minutes of kickboxing

Protein, indeed, is used for muscle building when it's converted to amino acids, but even excess protein can be converted into fat if it goes unused by muscles. Carbohydrates are used by your body's organs and systems for energy. Simple carbs (like sugary foods) are absorbed quickly, while complex carbs (like whole grains) are absorbed slowly. Those simple carbs lead to sharp spikes and then drops in glucose levels, which is why you feel the highs (and subsequent lows) from sugary snacks. Now, if there aren't sugars available for your body to use, your body will seek energy from fat. But if there's excess energy in any form, there's no place for those nutrients to go except to be converted into fat and stored throughout your body. Healthy fats—unsaturated fats found in olive oils, nuts, and fish—help keep you satisfied and play a role in keeping your arteries clear, and you need fat in your diet. (The more destructive fats—saturated and trans fats—are the ones you stay clear of.)

All of this means that you have to make portion control a reasonable part of your approach—even too much of the good foods can lead to fat storage. So the ideal equation for building a bikini body is reasonable portions of healthy foods. That ensures you get balanced nutrients, avoid the peaks and valleys of trying to eat simple carbs, and eat just enough to fuel your body, rather than store it as fat. So follow the portions guidelines I outlined in the last chapter and revolve your meals around these bikini-worthy BEACH foods.

B Body Buffers
Muscle-building proteins

As you'll see, building a little muscle is an essential part of the Bikini Body Diet program. The reason for that: Besides giving you that strong and sexy look, muscle also helps keep your metabolism revved so you burn more fat—in fact, it takes more calories for your body to maintain a pound of muscle than it does to maintain a pound of fat. It also helps you better navigate the rigors of life and prevent injuries. And it looks *gooooood*. You'll build toned muscle in this workout, but your muscle is like anything else that needs to grow and thrive—it needs fuel. That fuel comes in the form of protein, which is the building block of muscle. (This doesn't mean you're automatically going to start developing bodybuilder-like biceps if you start resistance training and increasing your protein.) The other big advantage of making sure you have protein is that protein helps keep you satiated so that you fend off urges to gnaw on cheese-flavored this or barbecue-flavored that at, oh, about 4:30 p.m.

8 pigs in a blanket
620 calories

YOU ATE IT?
NEGATE IT!
90 minutes of snow shoveling

Not all proteins are created equal, however, and there's plenty of damage that you can do with fatty sources of it (such as some cuts of red meat that are high in saturated fat; hello, rib eye). So you'll focus your meals around lean sources of protein—foods that are packed with it but don't have a lot of saturated fat. That means eggs, fish, chicken, turkey, and even some lean red meats.

Though it's not always possible, try to fit protein into your first meal of the day. (That's where eggs come in so handy.) Consider a recent study in the *American Journal of Clinical Nutrition*, which found that a high-protein breakfast can change body signals associated with food intake—meaning that protein helps improve satiety and reduce, as they say, "food motivation." And a 2012 study review from the Netherlands published in the *British Journal of Nutrition* showed that protein helps contribute to weight loss through a number of mechanisms, including increasing satiety. The review also concluded that protein helps lower blood pressure, while some research pointed to the conclusion that a low-protein intake can contribute to weight gain. A 2013 study in the *American Journal of Clinical Nutrition* found that having breakfast changed hormonal signals that control appetite, but that only a high-protein breakfast led to changes in signals that led to reductions in nighttime snacking. And researchers at Hebrew University of Jerusalem found that dieters who ate more protein than carbohydrates at breakfast and lunch and reversed the ratio at dinner lost more weight (26 pounds compared to 20) and felt more satiated than those who didn't.

Now, if you're one of those folks who's afraid to eat eggs because you think it leads to higher cholesterol, consider a couple of studies: A 2013 study in the *British Medical Journal* found that higher consumption of eggs is not associated with an increased risk of coronary heart disease or stroke, while a 2012 review of studies showed a number of trials in which there was no negative relationship between eggs and cardiovascular health.

What's great about proteins is there are so many of them. You can combine the BEACH foods, including your healthy proteins, carbs, and vegetables, to make delicious, power-packed meals. A veggie omelet, a chicken stir-fry, a beef and bean burrito... Filling, fulfilling, and fun!

MY WORKOUT PLAYLIST

Jillian Michaels

Nicki Minaj, "Moment 4 Life"

Lil' Wayne, "6/7"

Kanye West, "Hell of a Life"

Eminem, "White Trash Party"

Chris Brown, "I Can Transform Ya"

Kairo Kingdom, "One Two"

Avicii and Sebastien Drums, "My Feelings for You"

Alex Clare, "Too Close"

Skrillex, "Bangarang"

MIA, "Bad Girls"

The Bikini Body Diet

But when you ask the expert advisors, doctors, weight-loss coaches, and celebrities which types of protein they most favor, the same two answers pop up again and again: Healthy fish and eggs. Tuna, for example, has omega-3 fatty acids, which stimulate the production of leptin, a hormone that increases the feeling of fullness (so you stop eating sooner than you normally might). Salmon and mackerel are also good sources. Those fatty acids have other protective elements, too. Swedish researchers found that eating three servings of seafood a week can lower stroke risk by 16 percent, and one study published in the *Journal of the American Dietetic Association* found that people who consumed the most omega-3 fatty acids were 20 percent less likely to have gum disease than those who consumed the least (this is important because higher risk of gum disease is associated with higher risk of heart disease).

Quizno's Regular Tuna-Melt Sub
1,420 calories
YOU ATE IT? NEGATE IT!
2.5 hours of cross-country skiing

While more and more women are becoming educated about the benefits of protein, many women unintentionally ignore protein as a key component to their diet. According to research from the U.S. Department of Agriculture, 30 percent of women don't get enough protein. But it's essential. And vegetarians need to make a concerted effort to include beans and dairy products to make sure they're getting regular servings of protein every day. Nonfat Greek yogurt can also be an excellent source of protein that has additional health benefits. In a Tufts University study, researchers found that regular yogurt eaters were 31 percent less likely to develop hypertension.

A study in the journal *PLoS One* found that when people lowered their protein intake by as little as 5 percent and made up the difference with carbohydrate-rich foods, they ate an additional 260 calories a day. That adds up quickly. And it also shows you the potential satiating power of a protein-packed meal. In fact, Danish researchers found that dieters who got up to a quarter of their calories from protein lost an average of 22 pounds in just a few months. Don't skimp.

YOUR BEST BETS:

Nonfat Greek yogurt

Eggs

Chicken

Turkey

Sirloin (red meats with "loin" are lean choices)

Pork tenderloin

Tuna

Salmon

Mahi mahi

Shrimp

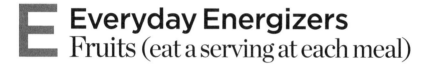

E Everyday Energizers
Fruits (eat a serving at each meal)

There's a reason why food marketers love to steal the label of "fruit" and tag it onto foods that are nowhere close to being nutritionally similar (think Froot Loops, Fruit Roll-Ups, Juicy Fruit, Fruity Pebbles). That's because they know that the word *fruit* just oozes with messages of healthfulness. If it says "fruit," it's gotta be good for you! Well, in most cases, that's true only if it's real fruit. (If only real fruit came with such strong marketing lingo.)

Along with vegetables, fruits should make up the largest portions on your plate, because they're packed with nutrients, like antioxidants and fiber (to keep you full). And the health benefits are simply massive. So much research points to fruits being strong disease-preventers. A 2012 study published in the *Journal of the Academy of Nutrition and Dietetics* that studied overweight women found that after four years, eating more produce was one of the important predictors of weight loss.

Pick a fruit; name the benefit. A couple of examples: Research from the Harvard School of Public Health found that eating two half-cup servings of blueberries can lower your risk of type 2 diabetes by as much as 23 percent. And grapefruit contains naringenin, an antioxidant that has been shown to help your body use insulin more efficiently, keeping your blood sugar in check and improving your calorie burn.

Plus, potassium—found in lots of produce, such as bananas and avocados—can have protective effects. A study in the *Archives of Internal Medicine* found that people who consumed the least potassium (and the most sodium) were more likely to die from cardiovascular disease than those who consumed the most potassium and least sodium. And fruits are key from a beauty standpoint, too. A study published in the journal *Evolution and Human Behavior* found that people who ate the most fruits and vegetables had healthier-looking skin than those who ate the least amount of produce.

Another advantage to hitting the produce aisle: Fruits also play a role in satisfaction. They can be your new source of sweetness to help satisfy cravings you may have. Pretty soon, you'll find that the natural sweetness in fruits is plenty decadent; they also serve as the sweeteners in some of the power-packed Bikini Body Diet juices. If you're a hardcore sweets addict, it may seem hard to believe, but it's possible to retrain your taste buds. (When you give up sugared sweets for the 7-Day Super Slimdown, you'll notice that jump-started in short order.)

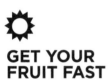

GET YOUR FRUIT FAST

Quick tip: Sign up for a community supported agricultural program (CSA): For a membership fee (sometimes around $20 a week), you'll get batches of fruits and vegetables from a local farm. It'll give you incentive to integrate increasing amounts of produce into your meals, and inspire you to try new things—and try unfamiliar produce, as well.

Fruit is also a great substitute for dessert, a nice bulker to homemade smoothies, and even a good way to add a little sweetness to a meal (hello, pineapple chicken!). There's no secret here: Eat more fruit and vary your choices so you're getting the most diverse nutritional benefits possible. And while you're at it, don't forget to get the blues: While blue and purple fruits make up only 3 percent of the average American's produce intake, they have huge benefits should be consumed regularly. A study from the *American Journal of Lifestyle Medicine* showed that adults who ate one or more servings a day of plums and blueberries had a lower Body Mass Index as well as other positive health indicators, such as lower levels of certain risk factors for cardiovascular disease.

Finally, don't forget a few things that fall off a tree but aren't often thought of as fruits. Avocados, olives, and nuts (while the latter isn't technically a fruit) all fit here because of their whopping nutritional counts; they also come with monounsaturated fat, which helps reduce belly fat.

YOUR BEST BETS:

Apples	Grapes
Oranges	Kiwi
Berries (all)	Mango
Grapefruit	Papaya
Melons (all)	Avocado
Apricots	Tomatoes
Peaches	Olives
Pineapples	Nuts (pecans, walnuts, pine
Bananas	nuts, almonds, cashews,
Pears	pistachios)
Plums	

A All-U-Can-Eat Anchors
Vegetables (as much as you want)

As a child, maybe you hated to hear the motherhood mantra of "Eat your veggies." They simply weren't as fun as fries, right? But any of you now on the other end of the spectrum (imploring your children to do the same as your parents wanted you to do) know exactly why: Veggies are nutritional deities. They're filled with vitamins and minerals;

they're usually low in calories; and, despite how they're stereotyped, they can taste amazing.

It won't come as any surprise that increased vegetable consumption correlates with increased weight loss. And one study even found that people who ate a dish made with pureed vegetables (like carrots, squash, and cauliflower) ate up to 360 fewer calories a day. (Gives you some good ideas: Put spinach into meatloaf, sweet potatoes into pancakes, or pureed veggies into a burger.)

It's a bottom line that will always affect your bottom line: More vegetables = a better body. The most bang for your nutritional buck will come from the leafy green water-based ones, such as spinach and kale, as well as the cruciferous ones like broccoli and cauliflower; both groups offer high nutrient and fiber content for minimal caloric investment.

MY WORKOUT PLAYLIST

Jordin Sparks

Rascal Flatts, "Fast Cars and Freedom"

Jay-Z and Kanye West, "Otis"

Jason Derulo, "Givin' Up"

Adele, "Rolling in the Deep"

Black Eyed Peas, "Rock That Body"

The evidence is clear that vegetables assist with weight loss and the health problems that come with being overweight, such as high blood pressure. Perhaps biggest of all: According to a study in the *Archives of Internal Medicine*, people who ate the most vegetables rich in alpha-carotene (found in leafy greens, broccoli, and carrots) had a 39 percent lower risk of premature death than those who ate the least. Many of the benefits of vegetables are attributed to their antioxidant content, which helps combat destructive chemical processes in the body.

For example, a 2011 study in the *Journal of the American Dietetic Association* followed more than 800 people for five years, and increased intake of fruits and vegetables was associated with the most weight lost. A Brazilian study published in the journal *Nutrition & Research* showed that an increased intake of fruits and vegetables correlated with a decrease in weight. And a 2012 Australian study published in the journal *Free Radical Biology and Medicine* looked at the effects of spinach and apples on the function of blood flow, and it found that both helped improved artery dilation—which helps improve circulation and reduces blood pressure. A study published in the *British Medical Journal* found that eating one and a half extra servings of green vegetables a day can help reduce the risk of developing type 2 diabetes—a condition associated with being overweight—by 14 percent.

But the advantages don't end there. After all, having a bikini body is also about having a healthy body—for a long time. An Italian study published in the *Journal of Agricultural Food and Chemistry* found that vegetables like mushrooms, onions, white cabbage, and yellow bell peppers reduced free radicals, which are associated with cancer; and a 2011 study in the *Journal of the American Dietetic Association* concluded that the risk of colon cancer was significantly decreased among those who ate yellow vegetables like squash. Also, a 2012 Japanese study found that those women who did not have daily green and yellow vegetables had a fivefold higher risk of low bone mass compared to those who had them daily. (Thinner women can be at higher risk of low bone mass, so

Be the Ultimate Smoothie Maker

The fastest and easiest way to make and eat a super-nutritious meal is just a push of the (blender) button away. Smoothies—which can fulfill any dietary role from breakfast to side beverage to healthy dessert—can be packed with nutritious ingredients to turbocharge your nutrition. But careful now, you can quickly add in a lot of calories and turn your smoothie into a shake. Below, guidelines for creating a power-packed smoothie:

✳ Use four ounces of skim, soy, or almond milk. That will give you protein. You can also mix in four ounces of nonfat Greek yogurt.

✳ Add in a cup of fruit of your choice.

✳ Add two tablespoons of fiber-filled rolled oats or a tablespoon of chia seeds. They'll make it thicker, more filling, and more nutritious!

✳ Flavor with cinnamon or cocoa powder to sweeten it up without a ton of calories.

✳ Sneak in leafy greens like spinach or kale, which won't change the flavor much but will help you get more nutrients.

that's important, especially as women get older.)

Beans belong in this category as well because they're packed with protein and fiber, so they are going to satisfy and help keep it at bay. Most beans are wonderful sources of nutrients (one notable exception being refried beans, which are often fried in lard), and, of course, as a staple in many vegetarians' menus, they can be prepared in, oh, about a zillion and a half ways.

Classified as both proteins and starchy vegetables, beans contain fiber, folate, and disease-fighting antioxidants. A 2012 study review in the *British Journal of Nutrition* found that beans have a positive impact in reducing the risk of certain diseases, such as cardiovascular disease and cancer. Another 2012 study in the same journal found that those who consumed a diet rich in beans, chickpeas, peas, and lentils saw their cholesterol drop by about 9 percent compared to those who didn't. And a 2012 Iranian study found that those people who consumed higher levels of legumes had the lowest risk factors for developing problems associated with metabolic syndrome, including high blood pressure, blood sugar, and cholesterol.

You'll see many of our recipes (especially our juices) in the next chapter have a strong vegetable base for all these reasons. If there's one category of truly "super" foods, vegetables would be it. They're low-cal, satisfying, and packed with properties that make your whole body healthier. If you have to keep one thing in mind during your journey, make it this: Fill half your plate with veggies and you've just about won the meal.

YOUR BEST BETS:

Broccoli	Squash
Spinach	Peppers
Asparagus	Cauliflower
Romaine lettuce	Cabbage
Kale	Brussels sprouts
Celery	Sweet potatoes
Carrots	Swiss chard

Collard greens

Cucumbers

Onions

Leeks

Beans (black, green, kidney,
navy, lima, garbanzo)

Peas

Lentils

C Crucial Carbs
Good grains (the healthy ones)

If there's one hot-button word in all of dieting, we can all pretty much agree on what it is: *Carbs*. All carbs, some carbs, no carbs, right carbs, wrong carbs, your carbs, my carbs, closet full of carbs... Oh my!

Well, here's the bottom line: There are a lot of bad, junky foods out there, and yes, many of them are very much carb-based. And that's one of the reasons why carbs have gotten such a bad rap, because it's not necessarily about the carbs, but about refined carbs: the simple sugars that have zero nutritional value and are so often associated with people putting on weight. So yes, there is such a thing as "good" carbs, and they're important for you to have as part of a balanced diet.

Cheese-flavored crackers
180 calories
per 1.25-oz bag
YOU ATE IT?
NEGATE IT!
26 minutes of leisurely bicycling

Whole grains (preferably foods made with 100% whole grains) are high in fiber, which will help slow your digestion, keep you full, and regulate your blood sugar levels. These good carbs help give and restore energy to your body; and along with lean protein and healthy fats, they serve as a major nutritional component to a good diet.

A 2010 New Zealand study published in the *Journal of the American College of Nutrition* found people who had four servings of whole-grain foods (as a substitute for more refined carbohydrates) lost an inch in waist size during the course of the study compared to those who didn't. And a 2012 Chinese study published in *Nutrition Journal* compared two groups—one who ate oatmeal daily for six weeks and one who ate noodles for six weeks. The study found that those who ate oatmeal had a greater decrease in cholesterol levels and waist circumference than the noodle-eating group.

A 2012 Tufts University study published in the *Journal of Nutrition* looked at markers of a substance called plasma alkylresorcinols, which is tied to the intake of whole grains. Researchers found that those with the highest markers of the substance had a lower Body Mass Index (a good thing). And a 2012 Japanese study published in the same journal found that those who had diets consisting of whole grains, compared to those who had diets with refined flour, had a decrease in body fat; and the refined-flour group also experienced increases in total cholesterol and LDL (the bad kind), while the whole-grain group did not.

Fiber is one of the key components at work here—for one, because it helps you feel full. A 2011 study published in the journal *Physiology & Behavior* found that a whole-grain breakfast resulted in a higher amount of satiety and less hunger and desire to eat after four hours compared to those who ate refined flour during breakfast.

But the effects aren't just about losing weight; they are also about having good health for the long run. A study in the *Archives of Internal Medicine* found that women who ate 26 grams of fiber a day lowered their risk of dying from cardiovascular, infectious, and respiratory diseases by up to 59 percent compared to those who ate just 11 grams of fiber. A 2013 study in the *Annals of Epidemiology* looked at more than 70,000 women who developed type 2 diabetes. Researchers found that those with higher fiber intake had a lower risk of developing the disease, and they even suggested that small increases in whole grains can be beneficial (since the consumption of whole grains in this study population was around only one serving a day).

MY WORKOUT PLAYLIST

Marisa Miller

Bloc Party, "One Month Off"

Michael Jackson, "Wanna Be Startin' Something"

Jay-Z, "Dirt Off Your Shoulder"

Linkin Park, "Bleed It Out"

Guns N' Roses, "Welcome to the Jungle"

In addition, a 2012 study in the *American Journal of Clinical Nutrition* found that those with low dietary fiber intake had a higher acceleration of arterial stiffness as they age (that's a bad thing when it comes to blood flow and cardiovascular issues, especially since they're associated with obesity). And a 2011 Italian review of studies concluded that whole grains are associated with a lower risk of developing diabetes, cardiovascular disease, and cancer. A small study from the *British Journal of Nutrition* found that whole grains had an effect on lowering blood pressure. Plus, whole grains contain magnesium (more on that on page 31 and to follow); a 2011 Serbian study found that dietary magnesium reduced the risk of coronary heart disease. And researchers in Scotland found that eating three daily servings of whole grains could cut risk of heart disease by 15 percent and chances of stroke by 25 percent. The rea-

Coffee Break

As long as you don't litter it with so many extras that it might as well be an ice-cream sundae, coffee is perfectly OK to have as part of your diet. In fact, more research seems to point to the health benefits of coffee:

✴ Women who drank more than three 8-ounce cups a day were **20 percent less likely to develop basal cell carcinoma**—the most common type of skin cancer—than those who drank less than one cup a month, according to a study presented at an American Association for Cancer Research conference. The benefits seem to be due to the inflammation-fighting antioxidants found in coffee.

✴ Because it's a stimulant, coffee is likely to make you **feel less stressed and more energized.** Some research shows that women who had four regular cups of coffee a day were 20 percent less likely to become depressed over a 10-year period than those who averaged one cup or less per week.

✴ Research shows that a compound in coffee works with caffeine to help **produce new brain cells** and strengthen connections between them, thus helping to ward off forms of dementia.

NOTE: Some women should cut down on coffee, especially if they have a high risk of osteoporosis or insomnia, have fibrocystic breasts (caffeine makes them more painful), or take any prescription medications that may interact with coffee or caffeine.

son: Refined flour is stripped of all the good stuff like fiber, magnesium, and other vitamins and minerals. So the whole-grain approach assures you get those good-for-you ingredients.

The major problem, of course, is that carbohydrates are unlike most other major categories of food. Most of us know what a vegetable looks like and even the looniest of folks can't argue that a French fry should count as a yellow vegetable. But with carbs, the area is grayer than a London sky, especially when you add in more marketing lingo: Even sugar cereals can be "made with whole grains," but that doesn't mean that they aren't packed with nutritionally bankrupt refined carbohydrates as well. Oatmeal is a carb. But so is white sugar.

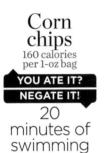

Corn chips
160 calories
per 1-oz bag

YOU ATE IT?
NEGATE IT!
20
minutes of
swimming

You want to get rid of sugars, refined carbohydrates, and high-fructose corn syrup (HFCS), a sweetener that has been linked to all kinds of diseases. Scientists believe that it simply acts differently in the body, negatively affecting hormonal reactions and other processes. In research published in the journal *Metabolism*, those who drank HFCS-sweetened drinks had higher fructose blood levels than if they'd consumed drinks containing sucrose (or regular table sugar). These elevated levels, researchers say, can lead to high blood pressure and insulin resistance.

So, on the Bikini Body Diet, you *will* eat carbs—and you *should* eat carbs for the weight-loss effect, satiety effect, and total-body health benefits. Here's how to make sure you're getting the right kinds:

For cereal, oatmeal (unsweetened) counts. And you can also enjoy unsweetened 100 percent puffed whole grains like wheat, rice, oats, barley, or corn. There are plenty of ways to add your own elements so that they have a little more zip if you want it. You can add cinnamon or even nuts, not just for crunch, but also to add protein and satiating healthy fats. If you prefer sweetness, add fresh or dried fruit instead of sugar; or sprinkle on some flaxseed to add in more fiber and omega-3 fats.

For breads and pastas, pick ones that are labeled "100% whole grain." That way, you know aren't getting refined flour, which has little nutritional value.

Choose brown rice over white (and definitely over fried!).

Popcorn (unbuttered) counts as a whole grain. One small study published in *Nutrition Journal* found that participants reported more satisfaction and less hunger when they ate popcorn compared to eating chips. And a study from the University of Scranton found that popcorn (prepared healthfully) can have twice as many of the antioxidants called polyphenols as apples and grapes. Choose air-popped kernels with low-cal additions, like some of the spices found in our next category of BEACH foods.

YOUR BEST BETS:

Oatmeal

100% Whole-grain bread

100% Whole-grain pasta

Brown rice

Cereal with 100% puffed whole grains

Quinoa (also high in protein)

Millet

Herbs and Spices
Flavor enhancers (that don't add sugar, sodium, or major calories)

One of the biggest complaints I hear from people who struggle with dieting is that they think that "being on a diet" means they have to sacrifice flavor. While, yes, there's no Doritos-flavored stir-fry here, that doesn't mean all of your meals have to taste like desk calendars. In fact, it's quite the opposite. And flavor is so important to having dietary success that I'm making it one of the five major groups in my BEACH foods.

As you progress, you'll likely use a combination of the recipes I've provided here, as well as developing your own recipes that utilize the BEACH foods. And when you do, I hope you'll say, "The 'H' with it! Let's come up

The Bikini Body Diet

with some new flavors." By experimenting with various herbs and spices, you'll likely find some combinations that taste decadent but aren't nutritionally destructive.

Though many of these spices do appear to have some weight-loss benefits, I'm not saying that a spoonful of a certain spice is the secret to weight loss. I am saying that what's at work here is something bigger: Because so many women "go off" their diets because they crave some flavor that's "banned" on their eating, the key is to make sure your meals are satisfying your tongue as well as your appetite. So try to find the spices, herbs, and flavors that do it for you so you don't have to have boiled chicken with lettuce every day. This way you'll be more likely to continue on the right path.

MY WORKOUT PLAYLIST

Malin Akerman

Nouvelle Vague, "This is Not a Love Song"

Radiohead, "Lotus Flower"

Led Zeppelin, "Whole Lotta Love"

Crookers, "Cooler Couleur"

Cary Ann Hearst, "Hell's Bells"

You can naturally boost flavor and nutrition in your Bikini Body Diet, with these fresh herbs and super-spices (they're also used throughout the sample recipes).

But you're also going to see some extraordinary health benefits as well, and that's another reason why herbs and other spices deserve their own special place of honor. For example:

FRESH HERBS

Basil: Contains vitamins A, C, K; and calcium, zinc, manganese, fiber, and iron.

Mint: Contains vitamins A, B6, C, E; and calcium. Also helps to soothe tummy aches.

Parsley: A true superfood, rich in disease-fighting antioxidants. Contains vitamins A, C, E, and K.

Rosemary: Contains iron and fiber. May help to improve circulation and aid in digestion.

SPICES

Cinnamon: Contains antioxidant properties, manganese, fiber, and calcium. Also aids in digestion. A study in Pakistan showed that daily ingestion of cinnamon can lower levels of cholesterol and blood sugar, and other studies show it may have an effect on lowering insulin (a hormone that promotes fat storage).

Chili powder: Helps fight inflammation; helps aid in cardiovascular health. May help to stimulate your metabolism.

Cayenne pepper: A Purdue University study found that people who sprinkled a half teaspoon of cayenne pepper on a bowl of tomato soup reported feeling less hungry and ate 70 fewer calories at their next meal.

Cumin: Contains antioxidant properties. Full of iron; helps aid in digestion.

Garlic powder: Contains manganese and vitamin B6; and has anti-bacterial, antiviral, and anti-inflammatory properties.

Ginger: Contains calcium, iron, magnesium. Aids in digestion and in lowering blood pressure. Helps improve feelings of nausea or an upset stomach. A small 2012 Columbia University study published in the journal *Metabolism* showed that subjects who consumed ginger had lower hunger and greater fullness than the control group.

Nutmeg: Has anti-inflammatory and antiviral properties.

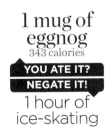

1 mug of
eggnog
343 calories
YOU ATE IT?
NEGATE IT!
1 hour of
ice-skating

CHAPTER 6

The Bikini Body Diet Meal Plan

Using the BEACH Foods in Quick and Healthy Recipes

So you're ready to get started? Good!

In this chapter, you'll learn exactly what and how to eat over the following weeks, with two distinct plans—one based on using the recipes that follow and one that's heavy in creating your own meals or ordering smartly on the fly, so you can stick to the plan whether you're eating in or out. A few things to keep in mind before we get started:

The Bikini Body Diet

Week One is the strictest. No alcohol, no sweets (except fruit), no additional sodium during the 7-Day Super Slimdown. Stick to three meals a day, with our homemade juices at two of them. It's a little tough, but the results will be dramatic. And it's only seven days.

Center all of your meals around the BEACH foods, with fruits and veggies taking up at least half your plate and lean proteins and healthy carbs taking up the rest.

Eat three times a day, with no snacking (though I do have a recipe for an excellent emergency snack if necessary).

Plan out your weekly meals and shop for ingredients ahead of time. Make as many Bikini Body Diet BEACH food meals yourself as you can. Research from the Fred Hutchinson Research Center in Seattle found that those who ate out for lunch at least once a week lost five fewer pounds than those who didn't go out as much. When you do reach for pre-packaged meals, however, make sure that the carbs the food contains are labeled 100% whole grains, and take a moment to survey the rest of the ingredient list. General rule: The fewer ingredients, the better. It might also help to know that those who say they look at nutrition labels weigh on average nine fewer pounds than those who don't. If you don't already read food labels, get in the habit.

WEEK 1 > 7-Day Super Slimdown: Classic

	SUNDAY	MONDAY	TUESDAY
MEAL 1	The Green Apple Juice	The Spicy Green Ginger Juice	The Cucumber Coconut Juice
MEAL 2	The Green Apple Juice	The Spicy Green Ginger Juice	The Cucumber Coconut Juice
MEAL 3	Salmon Niçoise Salad	Gluten-Free Garlic-Herb Pasta	Mini Bikini Veggie Burger

Note: Juices are best when consumed immediately after making them. If that's not possible, make enough for a double-batch, store cold, then stir vigorously before serving for Meal 2.

Beware the label hype. If you've ever bought a dress, brought it home, and the next day had a "What was I thinking?" shock, then you know that the heat of any shopping moment is a tough time to make smart decisions.

Well, the same goes for food shopping. But unlike a dress, which hangs in our closet for years, our poor food choices stick around in different ways—not always right in front of us. But they can stick around behind us, if you know what I mean.

Packaged foods are covered with words that seem to make them "healthier" than some other choice you might make. Words and phrases like "lower in fat" or "all natural" or "multigrain" sure sound appealing. Who wouldn't choose the all-natural multigrain product that's lower in fat?

Problem is, none of these words and phrases actually mean anything. The food that's "lower in fat" simply has less fat than the original version of the product—the "lower in fat" version may still be bulging with unnecessary calories. (And manufacturers often make up for the lack of fat with unhealthy doses of sugar and salt.) "All-natural?" So are crude oil and botulism, but I wouldn't pay to eat any of those. And "multigrain" means nothing more than "made from more than one grain"—it sounds healthy,

Recipe Version

WEDNESDAY	THURSDAY	FRIDAY	SATURDAY
The Sweet Carroty Green Juice	The Ultimate Pink Juice	Your favorite juice	Your favorite juice
The Sweet Carroty Green Juice	The Ultimate Pink Juice	Your favorite juice	Your favorite juice
Tomato and Mozzarella Panini Melt	Creamy Avocado and Orange Quinoa Salad	Ginger-Soy Marinated Chicken	Spicy Mahi Mahi Fish Tacos

The Bikini Body Diet

but if all of those various grains are stripped of their fiber and nutrients, you might as well be eating a teaspoon of pure sugar.

While the government has made some significant strides in getting nutrition information to the public—like requiring food packaging to carry nutrition labels, and large chain restaurants to post calorie counts—there's still so much room for trickery in our treats that reading the back labels (and ignoring the smiling models and cartoon characters

WEEK 1 > 7-Day Super Slimdown: Flexibil

	SUNDAY	MONDAY	TUESDAY
MEAL 1	Follow juice schedule from plan on pages 86 and 87		
MEAL 2			
MEAL 3	Create your own salad with protein of choice (dressing: 1 tbsp ea. olive oil + red wine vinegar)	Stir-fry, heavy on vegetables and protein of choice	4 ounces of chicken, brown rice, and vegetables of choice

Note: Juices are best when consumed immediately after making them. If that's not possible, make enough for a double-batch, store cold, then stir vigorously before serving for Meal 2.

SAMPLE WEEKS 2-6 > Flexibility

	SUNDAY	MONDAY	TUESDAY
MEAL 1	Sun-Dried Tomato, Basil, and Feta Frittata	Pineapple Coconut Smoothie Juice	The Green Apple Juice
MEAL 2	Create your own juice	Simple Tomato Soup	Simple Tomato Soup (leftovers)
MEAL 3	Tomato and Mozzarella Panini Melt	4 ounces of chicken, brown rice, and vegetables of choice	Create your own chili with ground turkey, black beans, tomato sauce, and vegetables

and amber waves of grains on the front) should be a regular habit of yours.

From pages 86 to 89, you'll see how the 7-Day Super Slimdown works, and how, if you take control of your food, you'll begin to see results quickly. Note that there's nary a packaged food on the list. Taking a little extra time in the evening or on the weekend can set you up with simple, healthy, bikini-friendly foods that will jump-start your weight loss—and get you the body you want!

ity Version

WEDNESDAY	THURSDAY	FRIDAY	SATURDAY
Follow juice schedule from plan on pages 86 and 87			
4 ounces of fish, black beans, and vegetables	Create your own salad	4 ounces of chicken, black beans, brown rice, and fresh salsa	Create your own chili with ground turkey, black beans, tomato sauce, and vegetables

Version

WEDNESDAY	THURSDAY	FRIDAY	SATURDAY
Create your own smoothie or juice	Eggs and fruit with 100% whole-wheat toast	Fresh Berry and Greek Yogurt Parfait	Omelet loaded with veggies, and a side of fruit
Chili (leftovers)	The Cucumber Coconut Juice	Lentil Kale Soup (leftovers)	Create your own juice
Create your own salad with protein of choice (dressing: 1 tbsp ea. olive oil + red wine vinegar)	Lentil Kale Soup	Mini Bikini Veggie Burger	Cheat meal

THE RECIPES

Juices

THE GREEN APPLE *Serves 1*

Ingredients:

- 1 Fuji apple*
- 1 bunch kale
- 1/2 lemon
- 2 celery stalks

Directions:

1. Place ingredients into a high-powered juicer, pour into a glass, and drink immediately.

~~~~~~

THE SPICY GREEN GINGER *Serves 1*

Ingredients:

- 2 tablespoons ginger (just break off a piece and toss it into the juicer, whole)
- 1/2 Fuji apple*
- 1/2 lemon
- 1 cup spinach leaves
- 1 bunch kale

Directions:

1. Place ingredients into a high-powered juicer, pour into a glass, and drink immediately.

For more sweetness add an extra 1/2 apple or a pinch of stevia.

THE CUCUMBER COCONUT *Serves 2*

Ingredients:

1/2 bunch kale

1 Fuji apple

1 large cucumber

1 cup coconut water

Directions:

1. Place ingredients into a high-powered juicer and add coconut water to blend. Pour into a glass and drink immediately.

THE SWEET CARROTY GREEN *Serves 1*

Ingredients:

6 cups spinach leaves

3 carrots

1/2 pear

Directions:

1. Place ingredients into a high-powered juicer, pour into a glass, and drink immediately.

THE ULTIMATE PINK *Serves 2*

Ingredients:

3 celery stalks

1 large cucumber

2 small beets (or half of one large)

1 tablespoon ginger (just break off a piece and toss it into the juicer, whole)

1/2 Fuji apple*

1 cup coconut water

Directions:

1. Place ingredients into a high-powered juicer and add the coconut water to blend. Pour into your glass and drink immediately.

Breakfast/Brunch

FRESH BERRY AND GREEK YOGURT PARFAIT

Serves 4

Ingredients:

- 1 cup nonfat Greek yogurt
- 1 cup fresh berries
  (a combination of blueberries,
  raspberries, or sliced strawberries)
- ¼ cup raw walnuts
- ¼ cup maple syrup or honey

Directions:

1. Place 2 tablespoons of Greek yogurt in an 8-ounce mason jar or cup. Top with 2 tablespoons of fresh mixed berries. Follow with 1 tablespoon of the walnuts.

2. Continue layering the parfait in this order for a total of two layers, finishing with walnuts on top. Drizzle the final layer of walnuts with 1 tablespoon of maple syrup or honey.

3. Repeat this process to assemble the remaining 3 parfaits; serve immediately.

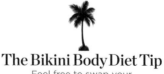

The Bikini Body Diet Tip

Feel free to swap your
favorite fruit into this recipe.
Peaches, mangoes,
or even pineapple
add delicious flavor.

SUN-DRIED TOMATO, BASIL, AND FETA FRITTATA

Serves 8

Ingredients:

  Nonstick cooking spray for pan

1 tablespoon extra-virgin olive oil

2 leeks, white and light green parts only, cut lengthwise, and thinly sliced into half-moons

2 garlic cloves, finely minced

½ cup oil-packed sun-dried tomatoes, drained and thinly sliced

8 eggs

1 teaspoon sea salt

½ teaspoon black pepper

½ cup fresh basil leaves, thinly sliced, plus more for garnish

2 tablespoons feta cheese crumbles

The Bikini Body Diet Tip

Frittatas are great for BLD. That's "breakfast, lunch, or dinner." Serve up this dish anytime. To lower the calorie count, cook with 4 whole eggs and 8 egg whites.

Directions:

1. Preheat the oven to 350 degrees. Lightly grease a 9-inch round pie plate with nonstick cooking spray.

2. Heat the olive oil in a small sauté pan over medium-low heat. Add the leeks to the pan and sauté until just softened, about 8 minutes. Reduce the heat to low, add garlic, and cook until leeks are tender and the moisture has evaporated, about 3 more minutes.

3. Place sautéed leeks and garlic evenly inside the pie plate along with the sun-dried tomatoes. Allow the mixture to cool for about 3 minutes.

4. In a medium bowl, whisk together the eggs, salt, and pepper.

5. Gently pour the egg mixture over the leeks and tomatoes. Fold in the basil.

6. Place the pie plate on the middle rack of the oven and bake for 30 minutes, or until the egg is set.

7. Remove the frittata from the oven and cool slightly. Cut into 8 servings. Top each with the crumbled feta and additional fresh basil, if desired. Serve immediately.

PINEAPPLE COCONUT SMOOTHIE

Serves 4

Ingredients:

- 2 cups frozen pineapple
- 1 large banana, frozen
- 1 tablespoon almond butter
- 2 tablespoons shredded coconut (optional)
- 2 cups coconut milk

Directions:

1. In a large blender, puree the pineapple, banana, almond butter*, shredded coconut (optional), and coconut milk until fully combined. Pour into 4 glasses and serve immediately.

*If needed, stop blender and carefully scrape sides with a spatula, then continue blending to combine.

The Bikini Body Diet Tip

Smoothies are perfect for the girl on the go. There's no better way to get your vitamins, calcium, and potassium in the morning with one quick blend. To cut calories, add more ice and less coconut shavings, or swap in coconut water for coconut milk.

EMERGENCY SNACK

Researchers from the University of California-Los Angeles, found that people who snacked on nuts, as part of a three-month diet, lost four more pounds than those who had carbohydrate-rich snacks. While the Bikini Body Diet plan calls for you to eliminate snacking, I also know that there are some times when you need to. If that's the case, reach for a handful of nuts, which are packed with protein and healthy fats to help stave off hunger. And if you're nuts for nuts, try the recipe on the next page for a snack with a kick. Keep your portion size to a handful, because nut calories can add up quickly.

ROASTED SOY-CHILI ALMONDS

Serves 6 (as a snack as needed)

Ingredients:

4 cups whole, raw almonds (about 1$\frac{1}{4}$ pounds)

1 tablespoon coconut oil

2 tablespoons low-sodium soy sauce

3 teaspoons chili powder

2 teaspoons garlic powder

$\frac{1}{2}$ teaspoon fine sea salt

Directions:

1. Preheat the oven to 350 degrees. Line two rimmed baking sheets with aluminum foil. Divide the almonds evenly between the two baking sheets and roast for approximately 8 minutes. Remove from the oven and cool slightly. Lower oven temperature to 300 degrees.

2. In a large mixing bowl, combine coconut oil, soy sauce, 2 teaspoons chili powder, and 1 teaspoon garlic powder. Add almonds and mix until well-coated and coconut oil has melted.

3. Place almonds back onto the baking sheets, return to the oven and roast for approximately 8 minutes more, stirring and rotating halfway through.

4. Remove from the oven and cool slightly. To finish, toss with the remaining chili powder, garlic powder, and sea salt. Store in an airtight container for up to 2 weeks.

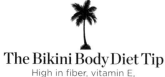

The Bikini Body Diet Tip

High in fiber, vitamin E, and magnesium, almonds are the perfect feel-good Bikini Body Diet snack. Bring these to the office or on your next road trip for a healthy snack.

Soups

SIMPLE TOMATO SOUP

Serves 4 to 6

Ingredients:

- 2 tablespoons extra-virgin olive oil
- 1 yellow onion, roughly chopped
- 4 garlic cloves, crushed
- 2 cans (28 ounces each) organic tomatoes, whole or crushed
- $\frac{1}{2}$ teaspoon sea salt
- 2 tablespoons fresh basil
- 2 cups low-sodium chicken stock
- Greek yogurt (optional)

Directions:

1. In a medium saucepan over medium heat, add the olive oil, onion, and garlic. Cook until soft and fragrant, approximately 15 minutes.

2. Add tomatoes and reduce heat to medium-low. Cook for 30 minutes. Add sea salt and 1 tablespoon basil, and cook for 5 more minutes. Remove from heat.

3. Carefully place the tomato mixture into a large food processor or heavy-duty blender. Slowly add the chicken stock while pulsing until fully pureed and smooth. Season with more sea salt to taste and serve. Top each bowl with the remaining fresh basil leaves and a dollop of Greek yogurt.

LENTIL KALE SOUP

Serves 4

Ingredients:

- 1 tablespoon extra-virgin olive oil
- ½ yellow onion, finely diced
- 2 carrots, quartered and sliced into ½-inch triangles
- 1 turnip, peeled and sliced into ½-inch pieces
- 1 bay leaf
- 8 cups low-sodium chicken or vegetable stock
- 1 cup lentils, rinsed
- ½ teaspoon sea salt, to taste
- 1 cup of thinly sliced Lacinato kale (optional)

Directions:

1. In a medium pot over medium-low heat, add the olive oil and onion, and sauté until just tender, approximately 4 to 5 minutes.

2. Add in the carrots, turnip, and bay leaf. Cook for 15 to 20 minutes, stirring occasionally, until onion is a deep brown color and carrots begin to soften.

3. Add ¼ cup of the stock and scrape the browned bits from the bottom of the pot. Add the rest of the stock and bring to a simmer. Stir in lentils and cook for another 30 to 40 minutes or until the lentils are soft. Season with salt to taste and add kale to finish.

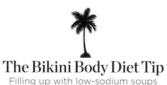

The Bikini Body Diet Tip

Filling up with low-sodium soups
is a great way to stay full longer
and can help whittle your waistline
while still satisfying
your hunger. Load soup with
plenty of nutrient-dense veggies (like
kale and spinach) and legumes.

CARROT GINGER SOUP

Serves 6

Ingredients:

- 2 tablespoons extra-virgin olive oil
- 1/2 yellow onion, finely chopped
- 2 pounds organic carrots, peeled and roughly chopped
- 2 garlic cloves, minced
- 2 tablespoons grated fresh ginger
- 1/4 cup orange juice
- 7 cups low-sodium vegetable stock
- 1/2 teaspoon sea salt, to taste

Directions:

1. In a large stockpot over medium heat, add olive oil and onions, and sauté just until soft and fragrant, approximately 8 minutes.

2. Add the carrots, garlic, and ginger and sauté until golden, stirring occasionally, approximately 20 minutes.

3. Add in the orange juice and vegetable stock. Bring to a simmer and cook until vegetables are soft, approximately 20 more minutes.

4. Carefully pour the mixture into a food processor or blender. Pulse until smooth. Season the soup with sea salt to taste.

5. Ladle into soup bowls and serve hot. Add a bit of extra ginger or orange zest to garnish.

Salads

CREAMY AVOCADO AND ORANGE QUINOA SALAD

Serves 4

Ingredients:

- 2 tablespoons extra-virgin olive oil
- 2 tablespoons balsamic vinegar
- 2 tablespoons orange juice (from a segmented orange)
- $1/4$ teaspoon sea salt
- $2^1/2$ cups cooked, cooled quinoa
- 1 orange, segmented
- $2^1/2$ cups arugula
- 1 ripe avocado, cut into 1-inch cubes
- 2 tablespoons crushed hazelnuts (optional)

Directions:

1. In a large mixing bowl, whisk together the olive oil, vinegar, orange juice, and sea salt.

2. Add the quinoa and orange segments to the mixing bowl and toss to coat in the vinaigrette.

3. Gently fold in the arugula and the avocado cubes. Divide among 4 plates and top with crushed hazelnuts, if desired.

SALMON NIÇOISE SALAD

Serves 4

Ingredients:

- 2 large eggs
- 1 cup fresh green beans, trimmed
- ½ teaspoon sea salt
- 1 bunch romaine lettuce, tough outer leaves removed, inner leaves thinly sliced crosswise
- ½ cup canned chickpeas, rinsed and drained
- 2 Roma tomatoes, thinly sliced lengthwise
- 1 can of high-quality canned salmon, drained
- 2 tablespoons red wine vinegar
- 1 tablespoon Dijon mustard
- 1 teaspoon honey
- 2 tablespoons extra-virgin olive oil

Directions:

1. Place eggs in a medium saucepan and cover with cool water. Bring to a boil, lower to a simmer for 3 minutes. Turn off the heat, cover, and set aside for 10 minutes. Remove the eggs and place in a bowl of cold water until cool enough to peel. Quarter each lengthwise and set aside.

2. Fill another medium saucepan with 1 inch of water. Place a steamer insert into the pot and bring the water to a boil over high heat. Add green beans and sprinkle with ¼ teaspoon of the sea salt. Reduce heat to low, cover, and steam until tender, about 6 to 8 minutes. Shock beans under cold water to stop the cooking, drain, and set aside.

3. Divide lettuce, chickpeas, and tomatoes among 4 shallow bowls. Top each serving with one quarter of the salmon and 2 egg quarters. Arrange the green beans on top.

4. In a small mixing bowl, whisk together the red wine vinegar, mustard, honey, and remaining ¼ teaspoon of salt. Slowly add in the olive oil, whisking constantly until well blended. Drizzle the dressing over each salad and serve.

Main Dishes

GLUTEN-FREE GARLIC-HERB PASTA

Serves 4

Ingredients:

1/4 cup extra-virgin olive oil

8 garlic cloves, thinly sliced

2 oregano sprigs, leaves removed from stems

1 cup dry white wine

1/2 cup finely chopped Italian parsley,
plus additional for garnish

1 teaspoon fresh basil leaves, julienned

1 teaspoon rosemary, finely chopped

1/4 teaspoon sea salt

1/2 pound gluten-free rice linguine

1 cup arugula

The Bikini Body Diet Tip

Cut your pasta in half and double the veggies, with spinach, sautéed kale, broccoli rabe, or asparagus. This will boost the fiber and vitamins A, C, and K; and reduce your carb intake.

Directions:

1. In a large pot, heat the olive oil over medium-low heat. Add garlic and oregano and sauté until a light-brown color appears, stirring frequently, approximately 8 to 10 minutes.

2. Reduce heat to low. Pour wine over the garlic and cook until the liquid reduces by one third. Remove from heat and stir in the parsley, basil, rosemary, and sea salt.

3. Meanwhile, cook the pasta according to package directions in a large pot of boiling, salted water.

4. When the pasta is al dente, strain and rinse with cold water. Toss the pasta gently in the garlic-herb sauce.

5. Using tongs, divide the pasta between 4 plates. Top with arugula and additional chopped parsley.

MINI BIKINI VEGGIE BURGER

Serves 4 to 6

Ingredients:

15 ounce can of chickpeas, drained

1/2 cup shallots, finely chopped

1 cup rolled oats

1/2 cup walnut pieces

1/2 teaspoon cumin

1 tablespoon lemon juice

2 tablespoons flat leaf parsley

2 tablespoons soy sauce

4 teaspoons extra-virgin olive oil, for frying the patties

The Bikini Body Diet Tip
Portion control is key and smaller portions can satisfy. Remember to eat only until you are just about full.

For serving:

Bibb lettuce leaves

Thinly sliced tomatoes

Avocado, halved and thinly sliced

Dijon mustard

Organic ketchup

Directions:

1. In a food processor combine chickpeas, shallots, oats, walnuts, cumin, lemon juice, parsley, and soy sauce and pulse for approximately 1 minute, until completely combined. Transfer to a medium bowl.

2. Shape the mixture into 6 patties, approximately $2\frac{1}{2}$ inches in diameter and $\frac{1}{2}$-inch thick.

3. In a medium sauté pan over medium heat, add 2 teaspoons of olive oil. Sear the patties in two batches, approximately 2 minutes on each side, until golden brown and heated through. Repeat with the remaining olive oil and patties.

4. To serve, place the patties on leaves of Bibb lettuce; top with tomato and avocado slices, a touch of Dijon mustard, and organic ketchup. Enjoy bun-less burger heaven.

TOMATO AND MOZZARELLA PANINI MELT

Serves 3

Ingredients:

2 tablespoons extra-virgin olive oil to toast and cook the panini

1 large vine-ripe tomato, or two small ones, thinly sliced

1 medium-size ball of fresh mozzarella, thinly sliced

$1/2$ cup of fresh basil leaves, loosely packed

6 slices of whole-wheat or Ezekiel grain bread, toasted with olive oil

Balsamic vinegar to taste

Directions:

1. Lightly brush the olive oil onto both sides of your bread, and toast in a medium nonstick pan over medium heat for approximately 2 to 3 minutes on each side.

2. On a clean work surface, add two tomato slices on top of the toasted bread, followed by two thin slices of mozzarella cheese and a few fresh basil leaves, with a touch of balsamic vinegar. Repeat, to make three sandwiches total.

3. In a medium sauté pan over medium heat, add a teaspoon of olive oil, place the assembled sandwiches in the pan.

4. To make a homemade panini press: Place another sauté pan faceup on the sandwiches, add a few heavy cans on top, and press down. Cook for approximately 2 to 3 minutes, flip, and repeat. Slice in half and serve with a side of Simple Tomato Soup (page 96).

GINGER-SOY MARINATED CHICKEN

Serves 4 to 6

Ingredients:

¼ cup low-sodium soy sauce

2 garlic cloves, finely minced

2 tablespoons white wine vinegar

1 tablespoon, finely grated ginger

1 tablespoon brown sugar

2 pounds free-range/antibiotic-free boneless, skinless chicken breasts

Directions:

1. In a medium mixing bowl, whisk together soy sauce, garlic, vinegar, ginger, and brown sugar and place into a resealable plastic bag or a container with a lid.

2. On a clean cutting board trim chicken breasts. Place the chicken in the bag with the marinade and make sure breasts are evenly coated. Marinate in the refrigerator for 25 to 30 minutes or overnight.

3. Preheat oven to 350 degrees. Spray a 9-by-13-inch glass baking dish with nonstick cooking spray.

4. Place the marinated chicken into the baking dish along with the marinade. Bake for approximately 30 to 35 minutes, or until an internal meat thermometer registers 165 degrees.

5. Remove from the oven and allow to rest 5 minutes. Thinly slice on the bias and serve over a bed of quinoa with a side of steamed vegetables.

~~~~~~~~~~~~~~~~~

PIZZA! PIZZA!
TIPS FOR MAKING IT HEALTHIER THAN EVER

✹ Choose a low-calorie crust made with whole grains. It will add more fiber to the meal and keep you fuller longer.

✹ Incorporate lean proteins like sliced chicken breast or pre-cooked spicy turkey sausage. Chop toppings into small pieces and spread evenly over the entire pizza, so you can boost the flavor of each bite.

✹ Lay off the sauce; jarred sauces can contain up to 550 milligrams of sodium per $1/2$ cup. Switch to fresh tomatoes and that sodium number plummets. Sprinkle with minced garlic and basil for added flavor.

✹ Use part-skim mozzarella rather than the whole-milk variety.

✹ Smother it with veggies!

~~~~~~~~~~~~~~~~~

SPICY MAHI MAHI FISH TACOS WITH ROASTED CORN SALSA

Serves 4

Ingredients:

For the Fish

- 1 tablespoon lime juice
- 1 tablespoon extra-virgin olive oil
- 1/2 teaspoon chili powder
- 1/4 teaspoon cumin
- 1/2 teaspoon sea salt
- 1 pound mahi mahi, cod, or tilapia
- 1 tablespoon coconut oil
- 8 small corn tortillas

For the Roasted Corn Salsa

- 1 cob roasted corn, shaved
- 1/2 yellow onion, finely diced
- 1 large cucumber, peeled and finely diced
- 1/4 teaspoon sea salt
- 2 tablespoons lime juice
- 1 avocado, finely diced

Directions:

1. In a medium mixing bowl, whisk together lime juice, olive oil, chili powder, cumin, and sea salt.

2. Cut the fish into bite-size pieces and add to the marinade, toss well to coat. Cover with plastic and place in the refrigerator for 20 to 30 minutes.

3. Meanwhile, make the corn salsa. In a large bowl, combine the corn, onion, cucumber, sea salt, and lime juice. Gently fold in avocado. Set aside.

4. Heat the coconut oil in a medium sauté pan over medium heat. When the pan is hot, add the fish and cook for approximately 7 minutes, until firm and opaque.

5. Place the cooked fish in warmed tortillas. Top with corn salsa and a squeeze of fresh lime.

Desserts

CINNAMON BAKED APPLES

Serves 4

Ingredients:

    Nonstick cooking spray

$\frac{1}{4}$ cup light or dark brown sugar

$\frac{1}{2}$ cup dried cranberries

$\frac{1}{4}$ teaspoon ground cinnamon

$\frac{1}{4}$ teaspoon nutmeg

 2 tablespoons water

 1 tablespoon lemon juice

 4 Red delicious or Fuji apples

 1 cup lemon sorbet or nonfat Greek yogurt

$\frac{1}{4}$ cup chopped walnuts, toasted (optional)

Directions:

1. Preheat the oven to 350 degrees. Spray a 9-by-13-inch glass baking dish with nonstick cooking spray.

2. In a small mixing bowl, combine sugar, cranberries, cinnamon, nutmeg, water, and lemon juice.

3. Cut a small slice off of the bottom of each apple so it can stand upright without wobbling. Using a paring knife, core the apples from the stem end leaving the bottom intact (remove about $\frac{3}{4}$ of the core). Use a vegetable peeler to remove 1 inch of the peel from the top of each apple.

4. Place apples in the baking dish and fill the cored centers with the seasoned cranberries, sprinkling any leftover cranberries over the top. Bake until the apples are soft and golden, 45 to 50 minutes. Remove from oven and set aside to cool slightly.

5. Add a few tablespoons of water to the syrup left in the baking dish to make it pourable. Drizzle the syrup over the top of each apple, and serve with lemon sorbet or nonfat Greek yogurt and toasted walnuts, if desired.

VANILLA AND FRESH MINT ICE CREAM

Serves 6 to 8

Ingredients:

- 2 cups skim milk
- 2 cups half and half
- 1/3 cup sugar
- 2 teaspoons corn starch
- 2 teaspoons organic vanilla extract
- 1 fresh vanilla bean, scraped (optional)
- 1/4 cup, fresh mint leaves, chiffonade (thinly sliced)

Directions:

1. In a medium mixing bowl add milk, half and half, sugar, and corn starch; whisk until combined. Place into the freezer for approximately 30 minutes.

2. Once chilled, place the mix into an ice cream maker and blend until thick, approximately 20 to 30 minutes. For a thicker consistency, place ice cream back into the freezer.

3. When ice cream is frozen to your preferred texture, transfer into a large mixing bowl and gently fold in the vanilla extract, vanilla bean (optional), and chopped mint; mix well. Place the ice cream back into the ice cream maker to mix for one last round, and then serve.*

Store for up to 3 weeks frozen in an airtight container.

CHAPTER 7

The Bikini Body Workout

This Easy Plan Will Get You in Shape in 6 Weeks

The fun thing about exercise is that there are a million things you can do to get fit. The downside: There are a million things you can do to get in shape. So, how do you know what's best, what works, and what the secret is to a bikini body?

Women often fall into the trap of doing only cardio-based workouts— like running, swimming, or sweating it out on an elliptical machine. And while cardio is tops for burning calories and also crucial for strengthening your heart and increasing your endurance, resistance training is

111

important, too. Incorporating strength training into your workouts will tone your trouble spots; and building sexy muscle (no bulk, we promise!) may even increase your daily calorie burn. That's why the Bikini Body Diet workout includes both types of exercise: cardio and strength training. After all, you don't just want to be slimmer; you also want sleek, sexy definition—it's the exclamation point on a swimsuit-ready physique.

In this program, you'll do some high-intensity cardio to blast calories and rev up your metabolism, and you'll also add strength moves to sculpt every major muscle group. Best of all, these strength workouts can be wrapped up in 30 minutes or less! We'll target areas like your abs, thighs, and butt, but also give you total-body workouts to make you strong all over. If you combine these sweat sessions with Bikini Body Diet nutrition principles, you'll slim down in record time. How fast? You'll see motivating results—a lift here, a sexy shape there—in just a couple of weeks. With that kind of kick-start, just imagine what you'll achieve in six weeks.

WEEKLY WORKOUT CALENDAR

	DAY 1	DAY 2	DAY 3
WEEK 1	Workout A See page 114 for details	Cardio See page 132 for details	OFF*
WEEK 2	Workout A	Cardio	Cardio
WEEK 3	Cardio	Workout A	OFF
WEEK 4	Workout B See page 124 for details	Cardio	Cardio
WEEK 5	Workout B	Cardio	Cardio
WEEK 6	Cardio	Workout B	Cardio

*For Off days, either do low-intensity exercise, like restorative yoga or walking, or don't work out. Your body needs recovery time to repair muscle and replenish energy stores. Skipping rest days may decrease your results and increase your injury risk.

WEEKLY WORKOUT CALENDAR

Make a copy of this schedule and post it somewhere you'll see frequently, like on your bedroom mirror or the refrigerator. Check off each workout as you do it and give yourself a reward for every week completed. (Try treating yourself to a mani-pedi or an exercise top, or downloading a new playlist.) Missed a session? Don't sweat it! Just do today's workout tomorrow.

TIP Schedule your workouts in your calendar as if they were important meetings and treat them as such. Allot 25 minutes (yes, that's it!) for Workouts A and B, and 20 to 60 minutes for cardio days.

DAY 4	DAY 5	DAY 6	DAY 7
Workout A	OFF	Cardio	OFF
OFF	Cardio	OFF	Workout A
Cardio	Workout A	Cardio	OFF
OFF	Workout B	Cardio	Cardio
Workout B	Cardio	Cardio	Cardio
Cardio	Workout B	Cardio	Success!

WORKOUT **A**

This routine sculpts sexy muscle in all the right places—flattening your abs, firming your butt, and toning your thighs. Plus, doing bursts of cardio between each move keeps your heart rate (read: calorie burn) high.

HOW IT WORKS Do 1 set of 12 to 15 reps of each move in order, performing 30 seconds of cardio (jump rope, do burpees, or march in place) between each exercise. Repeat the entire sequence once more. The last 2 reps of each set should be very challenging; if they're not, add resistance.

YOU'LL NEED A handled resistance tube, a pair of light (3 or 5 pounds) and heavy (8 or 10 pounds) dumbbells. (A weighted bar and ball, as well as a step or bench, are optional.)

1 TICK-TOCK SQUAT

Works biceps, butt, and legs

Stand on the center of a resistance tube with feet shoulder-width apart and hold an end in each hand at your sides, elbows bent 90 degrees and palms facing up. Squat, keeping your arms bent and chest high **A**. Rise up as you shift your weight onto your left foot and raise your right foot off the ground **B**. Try to maintain the same distance between feet. Return to starting position and switch legs on the next rep.

TIP Hold a light dumbbell in each hand (in addition to the band) to increase the difficulty.

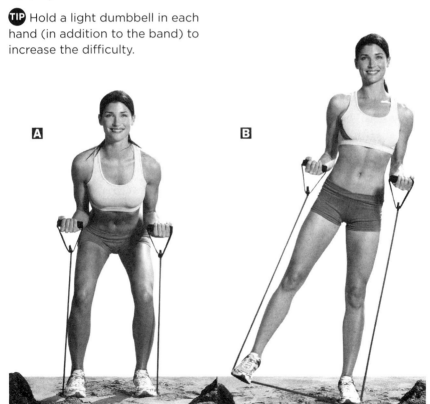

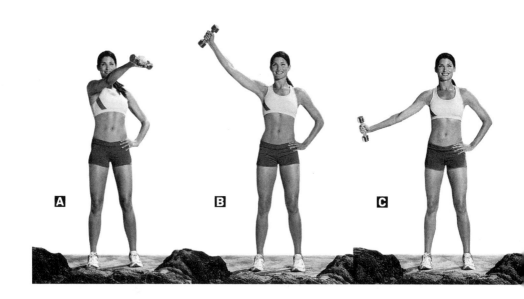

2 SINGLE-ARM ARC
Works shoulders and chest

Stand with feet shoulder-width apart and hold a light dumbbell in your right hand at shoulder level, palm facing away from you; place left hand on hip. Extend your right arm at shoulder height across your body to the left **A**, then raise it overhead, palm facing away from you. Move arm to the right **B** and slowly lower it in an arc **C** until it reaches your right hip. Return to starting position and repeat. Switch sides to complete set.

TIP Practice the motion without a weight first.

3 DUMBBELL CLEAN
Works shoulders, butt, and legs

Hold a heavy dumbbell in your right hand at shoulder level, palm facing toward you, and stand with feet wide and toes turned out, left hand on hip. Squat low **A**. Stand as you push the weight straight overhead, rotating your palm away from you and looking at the weight, extend left arm to your side **B**. Return to starting position; repeat. Switch arms halfway through set.

TIP Don't be afraid to use a heavy dumbbell for this exercise—your legs help power the weight overhead.

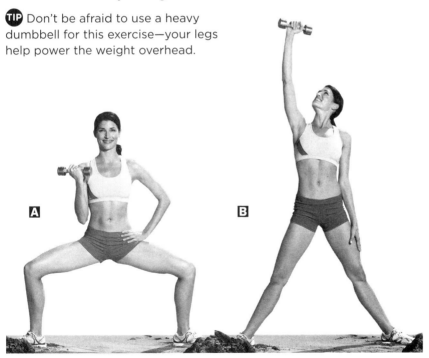

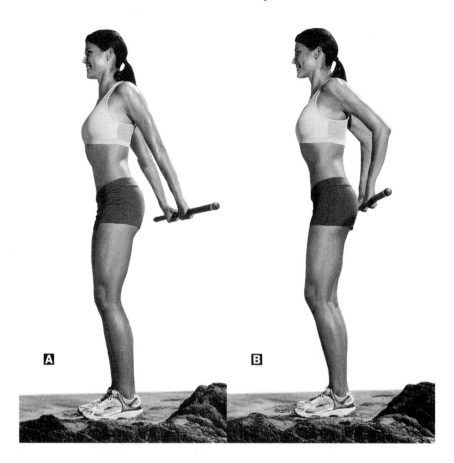

4 REAR-RAISE KICKBACK
Works triceps and upper back

Stand with your feet hip-width apart, knees slight bent, and hold a bar or two light dumbbells against your butt, arms shoulder-width apart and palms facing away from you. Lift the bar a foot away from your body **A**. Keeping your upper arms still, bend your elbows, bringing the bar toward your butt **B**. Straighten your arms to return to starting position.

TIP To help prevent your elbows from flailing outward, imagine you're squeezing a basketball between them.

5 SPLIT-STANCE ROW
Works biceps and back

Stand with your left foot on a step (or on the floor), knee bent, and right foot a stride's length behind it. Hold a heavy dumbbell in each hand, bend forward from your hips, and extend arms down, palms facing each other **A**. Bend your elbows back, drawing weights to your sides as you raise your torso **B**. Return to starting position and repeat; switch legs halfway through set.

TIP To help activate your back muscles, squeeze your shoulder blades together as you bend your elbows.

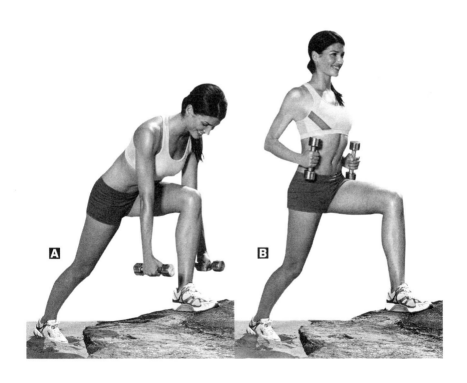

6 TABLETOP PRESS
Works chest and core

Hold a heavy dumbbell in each hand and lie faceup with your knees bent over your hips. Bend elbows 90 degrees and hold dumbbells at your sides, palms facing each other **A**. Press weights up over your chest **B**. Lower weights to starting position.

TIP If this is too challenging, do it with your feet flat on the ground.

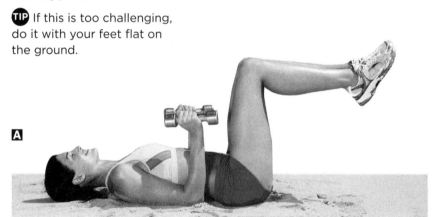

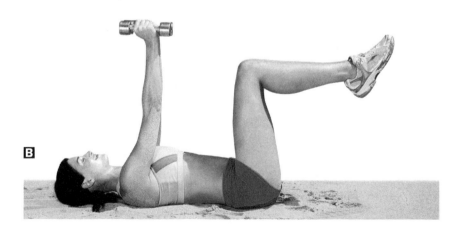

7 BUTT BLAST

Works core, butt, and hamstrings

Kneel on all fours with your wrists aligned under your shoulders and your knees under your hips, and place a light dumbbell behind your right knee. Raise your left arm to shoulder height in front of you, palm facing the ground **A**. (Beginners, keep both hands on the ground.) Lift your right thigh to hip height behind you, foot flexed **B**. Return to starting position and repeat. Switch sides to complete set.

TIP Pull your abs in tight to help activate your core and stabilize your body.

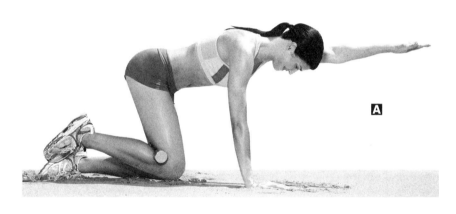

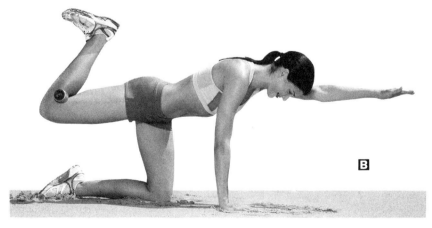

8 BICYCLE
Works abs

Lie faceup with your legs extended on the ground in front of you and hold a weighted ball or dumbbell over your chest, elbows bent out to your sides. (Beginners, skip the weight and place your hands behind your head.) Lift legs, head, and shoulders as you bend your right knee and rotate your left shoulder toward it **A**. Extend your right leg as you bend your left knee toward your chest and rotate your shoulder toward it **B** to complete 1 rep. Repeat.

TIP Focus on rotating your shoulder (not your elbow) toward your knee.

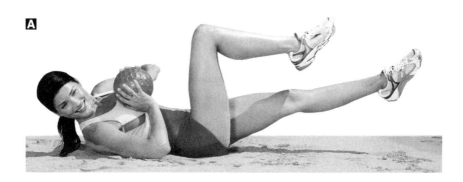

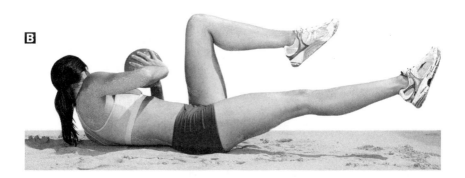

MAXIMIZE EVERY MINUTE OF YOUR WORKOUTS WITH THESE TIPS.

✳ Pick up the pace: Walking at 4.5 mph burns 66 percent more calories than going at 3.5 mph. Take short strides to increase speed.

✳ Add intervals: During any cardio workout, move as fast as you can, or increase the incline for 1 minute every 3 minutes to burn 10 percent more calories.

✳ Go heavy: The more a weight weighs, the more energy in takes to lift it (that equals a higher calorie burn and faster strength gains).

✳ Catch some air: At 9 calories burned per minute (compared to 3 or 4 for strength training), plyometric moves (like jumping) slim you down faster.

✳ Ditch the remote: Some research shows that you work at a lower intensity when you watch TV while doing cardio. Sub in tunes for the tube. A study in the *Journal of Science and Medicine* found that triathletes ran about 20 percent longer when they listened to tunes as compared to listening to nothing (and they had better results when the music matched their pace).

WORKOUT B

Varying your workouts, and continuing to challenge your body, is key to seeing results. To help you firm and burn, this plan combines strength moves with plyometrics—powerful exercises that often involve jumping and can burn 9 calories a minute. Be warned: This session is tough. But in just 21 minutes, you'll be done.

HOW IT WORKS Do each move in order for 1 minute. Repeat the entire circuit twice more.

YOU'LL NEED A pair of 5- to 8-pound dumbbells and a clock with a second hand (or your smartphone's stopwatch).

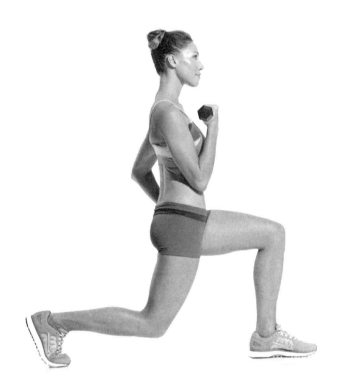

1 LUNGE CURL

Works biceps, butt, and legs

Stand with feet hip-width apart, holding a dumbbell in your right hand, your right arm extended at your side and palm facing forward; place left hand on hip. Lunge back with your right leg as you curl the weight toward your shoulder [shown]. Return to starting position. Switch sides after 30 seconds.

TIP To prevent yourself from bending forward, imagine a string pulling your head up toward the ceiling.

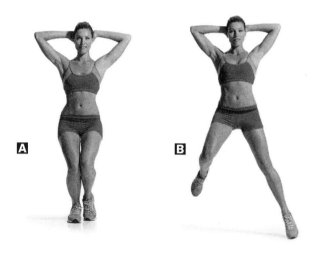

2 SIDE-SKATE
Works core, butt, and legs

Stand with your feet together, knees bent, and hands behind your head.
Lift your left heel **A** and jump to the left **B**, landing on left foot,
knees bent, and right foot raised. Jump back to starting position.
Continue, alternating sides.

TIP To decrease the intensity, step from side to side instead of jumping.

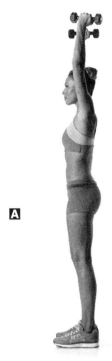

A

3 FLYWHEEL

Works triceps, shoulders, and core

Stand with feet hip-width apart, holding a dumbbell in each
hand overhead, arms extended and palms facing each other **A**.
Bend forward from your hips, knees slightly bent, as you lower your
arms until they're behind you **B**. Rise up to starting position.

TIP Focus on using your muscles—not momentum—to move your arms.

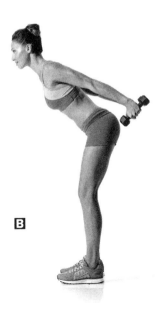

B

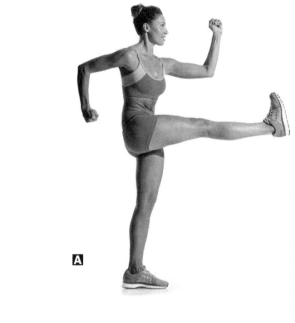

A

4 FRONT-REAR KICK
Works core, butt, and legs

Stand with feet together, elbows bent at your sides and your hands in fists. Kick your right leg straight out in front of you, foot flexed, as you bring your left arm forward and right arm back **A**. Bend forward from your hips, and kick your right leg behind you, switching arm positions **B**. Continue, alternating front and rear kicks. Switch sides after 30 seconds.

TIP If you start to lose your balance, slow down.

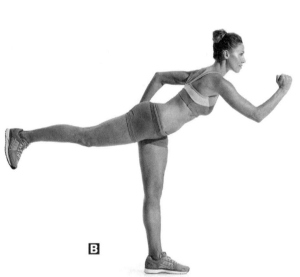

B

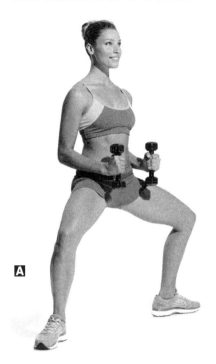

A

5 PUNCHING PLIÉ

Works shoulders, chest, butt, and legs

Stand with feet wide, toes turned out; hold a dumbbell in each hand with elbows bent at your sides and palms facing each other. Bend your knees **A**. Punch your left arm at a diagonal to the right as you rotate your palm toward the floor **B**. Return to starting position and repeat, this time punching with right arm. Continue, alternating arms each time.

TIP To make this move easier, do it without weights.

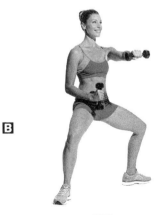

B

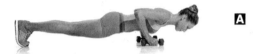

6 PUSHUP ROW

Works shoulders, chest, back, arms, and abs

Get in plank position, holding a dumbbell in each hand, palms facing each other. Bend your elbows, lowering your chest toward the floor **A**. Push up, then bend your right elbow straight back, drawing the weight toward your side **B**. Return to starting position and repeat, raising the left weight. Continue, alternating arms each time.

TIP To make this move easier, skip the pushups and perform only the rows.

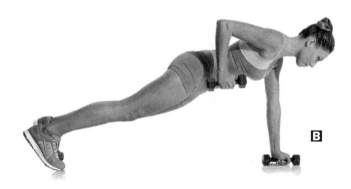

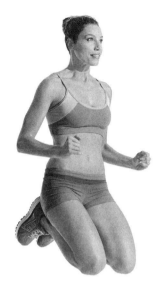

7 BUTT KICK
Works butt and legs

Stand with feet hip-width apart, elbows bent at your sides and hands in fists. Bend your knees and jump straight up, kicking your heels toward your butt [shown]. Land and immediately repeat.

TIP Challenge yourself every workout to complete more of these jumps in one minute.

Cardio Connection

While workouts A and B in this chapter get your heart rate up, adding some traditional aerobic exercise will help blast fat and keep your metabolism revved. That's why your weekly schedule includes plenty of cardio. The activity and amount of time are up to you, but aim to burn 250 to 500 calories during every session. Some ways to do it:

6 WAYS TO REACH YOUR CARDIO QUOTA *(calorie burn based on a 145-pound woman):*

Run for 20 minutes...BURN 250 calories

Do the "30-Minute Fat Blast" (below)...BURN 300 calories

Swim freestyle for half an hour...BURN 330 calories

Play tennis for 40 minutes...BURN 370 calories

Take a 45-minute group-cycling class...BURN 500 calories

30-MINUTE FAT BLAST

During this routine, you'll push yourself hard at a high intensity, recover, and repeat. Research shows that this type of workout (called high-intensity interval training, or HIIT) blasts more calories in less time than exercising at a steady effort level. Try this routine on any cardio machine or outdoors.

TIME (mins)	WHAT TO DO	RPE*
0-4	Warm up at an easy intensity	4
4-9	Increase intensity (up the speed, incline, or both) to moderate	6
9-10	Increase intensity to hard	7
10-11	Increase intensity to very hard	8
11-15	Return to moderate	6
15-21	Repeat minutes 9-15	5-8
21-22	Increase intensity to very hard	8
22-26	Return to moderate	5
26-30	Cool down	3-4

CLEAN UP YOUR RUNNING FORM

It makes all the difference in the world to use proper technique—you'll run faster, stay injury-free, and get the most out of every run.

✻ Look 5 to 10 feet in front of you, keep your head in line with your neck, and relax your shoulders.

✻ Hinge forward a little from your hips. (When going uphill, lean back slightly.)

✻ Take slow, steady, deep breaths to maintain control as you pick up speed.

✻ Your feet should strike directly under your body.

✻ Land on the ball of your foot and push off. If your heel hits first, it absorbs shock and acts like a break, slowing you down.

✻ If going downhill, try to kick your butt, which will help lengthen your stride. On an incline, kick back less.

✻ Keep your elbows bent 90 degrees and close to your body, and gently swing your arms forward and back.

*Rate of perceived exertion (RPE) is used to gauge your intensity in cardio workouts. Here is what the numbers indicate.

RPE 1–2	Very easy; you can converse with no effort
RPE 3	Easy; you can converse with almost no effort
RPE 4	Moderately easy; you can converse comfortably with little effort
RPE 5	Moderate; conversation requires some effort
RPE 6	Moderately difficult; conversation requires quite a bit of effort
RPE 7	Difficult; conversation requires a lot of effort
RPE 8	Very difficult; conversation requires maximum effort
RPE 9–10	Peak effort; no-talking zone

CHAPTER 8

Tone Your Trouble Zones

The Bikini Body Diet Belly, Butt & Thighs Workout

The bikini means many things to many people, but if I had to boil it down to one thing, it might be this: No secrets.

It covers what it needs to cover, and that's it. Which is wonderful—if you're feeling confident, sexy, and sleek. It can also be horrific if you're not in that place. I hope that you've already discovered the secret to no

The Bikini Body Diet

secrets—it's a combination of the right eating and exercise plans. But burning fat is only one element of this plan: By firming up particular body parts, you'll look better and feel better.

If you've been following the Bikini Body Diet workout program, your body is getting slimmer and sleeker—and you're feeling sexier—every day. But chances are you have a stubborn spot (or two) that could use a little extra sculpting. It's no surprise: Women store extra fat in the belly, butt, and thigh areas (thank you, Mother Nature), making them particularly challenging to reshape. While you can't spot-reduce—you need to eliminate fat all over to trim any area—you *can* spot sculpt. In this chapter, I show you eight moves that can target each of those three common problem areas. Combine the exercises with cardio on most days, and the Bikini Body Diet, and soon the nagging jiggle (and all the insecurities that come with it) will melt away.

HOW IT WORKS

If you're in the first three weeks (1–3) of the Bikini Body Diet workout program and you want to focus on your...

ABS > Before or after every cardio workout: Do 1 set of 15 reps of *two* of the abs exercises; choose a different pair every session.

BUTT > Before or after every cardio workout: Do 1 set of 15 reps of *two* of the butt exercises; choose a different pair every session.

THIGHS > Before or after every cardio workout: Do 1 set of 15 reps of *two* of the thighs exercises; choose a different pair every session.

ALL THREE TROUBLE ZONES > Before or after every cardio workout: Do 1 set of 15 reps of *an exercise from each trouble-zone workout* (1 abs move, 1 butt move, 1 thigh move); choose different exercises every session.

If you're in the second three weeks (4–6) of the Bikini Body Diet workout program and want to focus on your...

ABS > On Days 3 and 6 (before or after your cardio workout): Do 2 sets of 10 reps of *two* of the abs exercises; choose a different pair every session.

BUTT > On Days 3 and 6 (before or after your cardio workout): Do 2 sets of 10 reps of *two* of the butt exercises; choose a different pair every session.

THIGHS > On Days 3 and 6 (before or after your cardio workout): Do 2 sets of 10 reps of *two* of the thighs exercises; choose a different pair every session.

ALL THREE TROUBLE ZONES > On Days 3 and 6 (before or after your cardio workout): Do 2 sets of 10 reps of *an exercise from each trouble zone workout* (1 abs move, 1 butt move, 1 thigh move); choose different exercises every session.

If you've completed the Bikini Body Diet workout program, use the moves in this chapter to create several different trouble-zone toning workouts. Here's how.

To target one trouble spot... > Twice a week: Do 2 sets of 10 reps of *four of the exercises from one of the trouble-zone plans;* mix up the moves every session.

To target all three trouble zones... > Twice a week: Do 2 sets of 10 reps of *two exercises from each trouble-zone workout* (2 abs moves, 2 butt moves, and 2 thigh moves); choose different exercises every session.

TARGET: Abs

The secret to firming your abs fast (so you can show them off asap) is to crank up the intensity. These exercises do it by either adding resistance, challenging your coordination, or both. The result: You'll work harder than you would during an ordinary crunch and hit all your middle muscles, scoring sexy definition stat!

YOU'LL NEED A 3- to 6-pound medicine ball, a pair of 3- or 5-pound dumbbells, a stability ball, and a resistance band. (A mat is optional.)

ROPE CLIMB

Lie faceup with your knees bent and feet flat on the ground. Bend your arms and tuck your elbows close to your sides, about an inch off the ground; make loose fists with your hands. Raise your head and shoulder blades while reaching your left arm slightly to the right and up, extending your fingers as if you were reaching for a rope to pull it down [shown]. Lower your left arm and reach with your right arm while you rotate slightly to the left to complete 1 rep.

TIP Imagine the rope is dangling over the center of your chest—that's the direction you should reach.

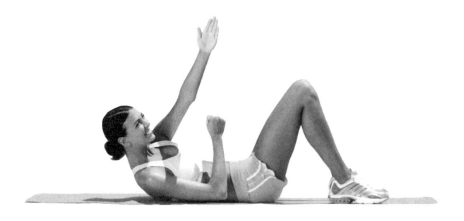

MEDICINE-BALL DOUBLE CRUNCH

Lie faceup with your knees bent over your hips and squeeze a medicine ball between your calves and upper thighs. (If you don't have a medicine ball, do the move without weight.) Place hands behind your head. Simultaneously lift your head, shoulder blades, and hips [shown]. Lower to starting position.

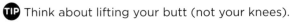 Think about lifting your butt (not your knees).

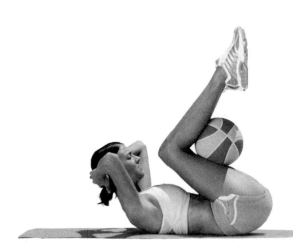

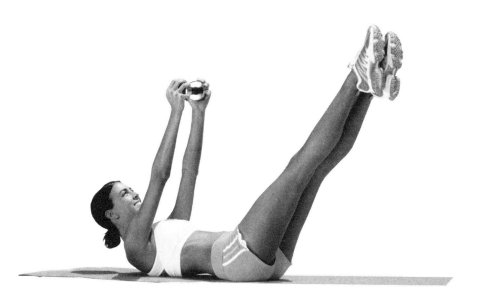

PIKE PRESS-UP

Hold a dumbbell with both hands and lie faceup, legs extended at a 45-degree angle off the ground. Extend arms straight up over your chest. Lift your head and shoulder blades, pressing dumbbell straight up [shown]. Lower to starting position.

TIP To make this move easier, extend your legs straight up over your hips; lowering your legs closer to the floor will make it more challenging.

DUMBBELL REACH

Hold a dumbbell in your left hand
and lie faceup with your knees
bent and feet flat on the ground.
Place your right hand on your belly
and extend your left arm straight
up in line with your shoulder.
Lift your head and shoulders as
you slightly draw your left shoulder
toward your right knee [shown].
Lower and repeat. Switch sides
to complete set.

TIP If your neck hurts, drop the weight
and place one hand behind your head
(and the other on your belly).

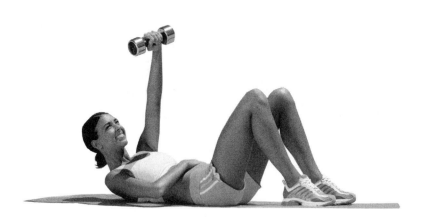

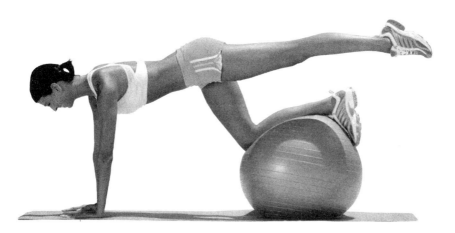

ONE-LEG KNEE-IN

Get in plank position with your shins on a stability ball. Raise your left leg a few inches. Press your right foot into the ball as you bend your right knee, rolling the ball toward your hands [shown]. Extend right leg to return to starting position and repeat. Switch sides to complete set.

TIP Don't have a stability ball? Hold plank position and draw one knee toward your chest, alternating knees each rep.

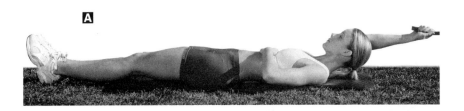

BAND PULL

Anchor one end of a resistance band around a sturdy object about a foot off the ground and grasp the other in your right hand. Lie faceup with your left hand on your belly and extend your right arm behind you; adjust your position so the band is taut **A**. Keeping your right arm next to your head, curl your shoulder blades off the ground **B**. Hold for 1 count, then slowly lower to start position and repeat. Switch sides to complete set.

TIP If your neck feels strained, place your free hand behind your head to support it.

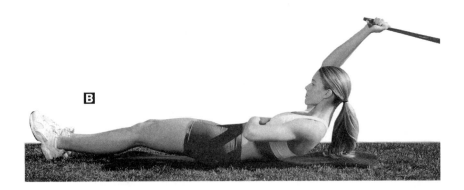

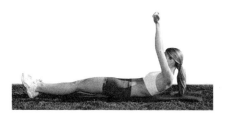

A

DUMBBELL ROLL-UP

Hold a dumbbell in each hand and lie faceup, arms extended over your chest, palms facing forward. Keeping arms straight up, slowly raise your upper body **A** until your torso is perpendicular to the ground **B**. Roll down to starting position.

TIP Move as slowly as you can, curling one vertebra at a time up and then down.

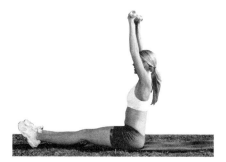

B

BALL TWIST

Hold one end of a dumbbell in both hands and lie with your shoulders centered on a stability ball. Place feet shoulder-width apart on the ground and extend arms over your chest so dumbbell is vertical. Lift hips so your body is straight from your head to knees **A**. Keeping arms straight and hips raised, rotate your torso to the left (ball will move under you) and lower weight until arms are parallel to the ground and left shoulder is centered on the ball **B**. Return to starting position and repeat to the right side to complete 1 rep.

TIP Start the motion in the middle of your abs, and focus on using your belly to do all the work.

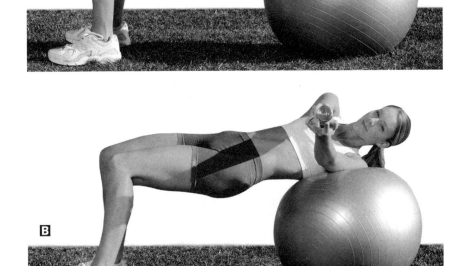

Get Wobbly

Using a stability ball, balance disc,
or Bosu activates more muscle fibers
in your midsection than performing
the same exercise on the floor.

TARGET: Butt

Booty confidence: It's what allows a woman to strut her stuff in a bikini sans board shorts or a sarong—and the moves here will help you get it. These exercises work your glutes to their limit, helping to reshape your rear. Plus, they strengthen your hamstrings (the muscles along the back of your thighs)—the stronger they are, the more lifted your butt will be.

YOU'LL NEED A 2- to 6-pound medicine ball, a pair of 5- to 8-pound dumbbells, and a resistance band.

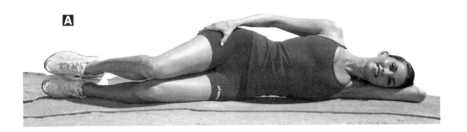

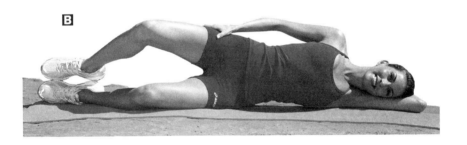

CLAM

Lie on your left side, head on your left arm, and bend your knees in front of you so your feet are in line with your hips. Place your right hand on your outer thigh **A**. Lift your right knee as high as you can without rocking back or separating your feet **B**. Lower and repeat. Switch sides to complete set.

TIP To increase the challenge, tie a resistance band around your thighs.

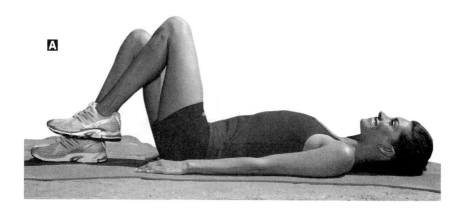

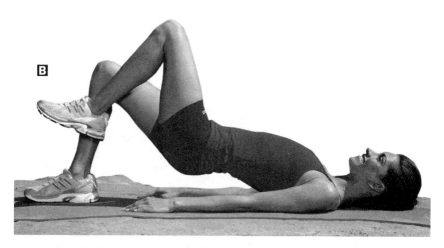

SINGLE-LEG BRIDGE

Lie faceup with your knees bent and your feet just
in front of your hips. Extend your arms at your sides,
palms on the ground. Lift your left foot a few inches **A**.
Press your right foot into the ground and lift your hips
several inches **B**. Then lower your hips until they almost
reach the ground, keeping your left foot raised,
and repeat. Switch sides to complete set.

TIP If this is too tough, do it with both feet on the ground.

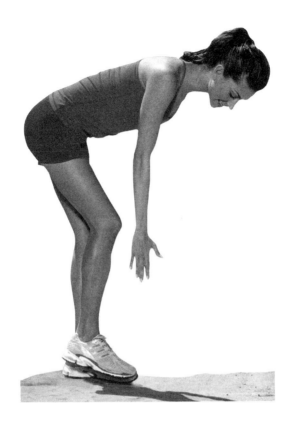

SINGLE-LEG TOUCHDOWN

Stand with your feet hip-width apart, arms extended at your sides. Lift your right foot an inch or so off the ground. Keeping your back straight (don't hunch or arch), bend over from the hips and reach your right arm toward left foot [shown]. Rise up and repeat. Switch sides to complete set.

TIP Stand on a pillow or balance disc to make this move more challenging.

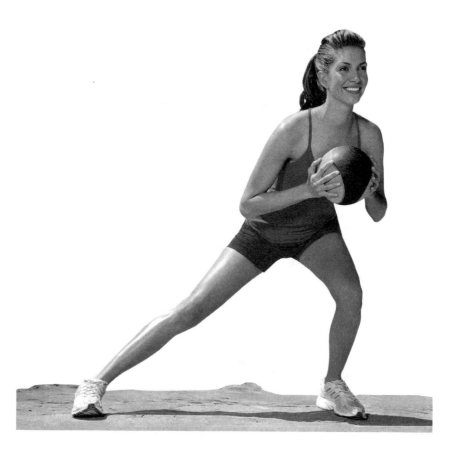

LATERAL LUNGE

Hold a medicine ball or dumbbell in both hands in front of your chest and stand with feet wide. Keeping your feet parallel, lunge to the left so your left hip is aligned with your left foot [shown]. Rise up to return to starting position, then repeat to the right to complete 1 rep.

TIP Push your hips back when you lunge, as if you were sitting down in a chair.

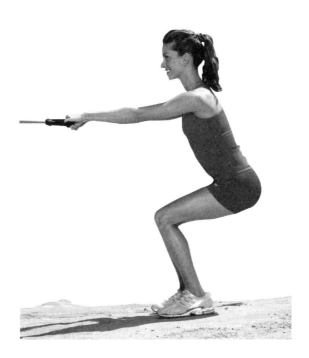

BAND SQUAT

Anchor the center of a resistance tube to a sturdy object at chest height or slightly lower and hold a handle in each hand. Stand with feet shoulder-width apart, arms extended in front of you, and lean back slightly. Squat [shown], then rise up to starting position.

TIP If it's difficult to balance, perform this move without the band or while holding the edge of a counter.

FLOOR DEADLIFT

Stand with feet hip-width apart and place a dumbbell on the floor, slightly in front and to the outside of each foot. Squat until your thighs are parallel to the floor, and pick up the weights. Push through your heels and keep your back straight as you stand up. Keeping your back straight and a slight bend in your knees, bend forward from your hips and the lower the weights [shown] back to the floor.

TIP Look forward, not down, as you lift and lower.

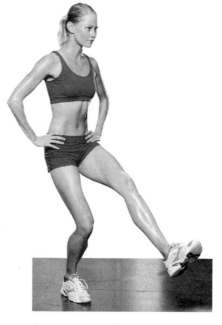

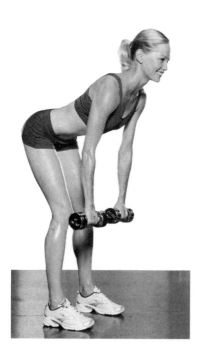

SINGLE-LEG SQUAT

Stand with feet shoulder-width apart and place your hands on your hips. Lift your left foot a few inches off the floor in front of you. Bend your right knee [shown], rise up, and repeat. Switch legs to complete set.

TIP Don't bend your knee more than 90 degrees.

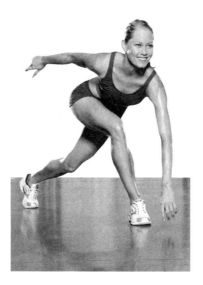

SPEED SKATER

Stand with feet together and lunge your left foot back and to the right as you reach your left hand toward your right foot [shown]. Hop to the left and repeat to complete 1 rep.

TIP To make this move easier, skip the hop and simply step from side to side.

TARGET: Thighs

High-cut bikini bottoms can help create the illusion of longer legs, but there's no fashion fix for thigh bulge. Thankfully these exercises solve the problem. They sculpt the muscles on the front, side, and back of your legs, so you can confidently hike up your hemline.

YOU'LL NEED A pair of 5- to 8-pound dumbbells, a step or bench, a resistance band, a stability ball or chair, a Pilates ball or playground ball, and a resistance tube or band.

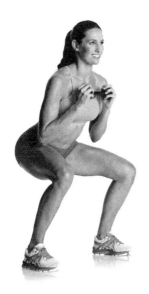

SQUAT JACK

Stand with your feet hip-width apart, and hold a dumbbell in front of your chest. Squat until your thighs are parallel to the floor. Staying in the squat, jump up, landing with feet wide [shown]. Jump back to starting position.

TIP The lower you are, the more challenging this move will be—try to keep your knees bent for the entire set.

CROSS LUNGE

Stand with your feet wide and parallel, holding a dumbbell in each hand on your hips, elbows pointing behind you. Lunge to the left as you place the right dumbbell on the floor in front of left toes [shown]. Lunge to the right and place the left weight in front of right toes. Lunge to the left again and pick up the weight with your right hand; lunge to the right to pick up the weight with your left hand to complete 1 rep.

TIP When you lunge, imagine pressing your foot, knee, and outer thigh against a wall.

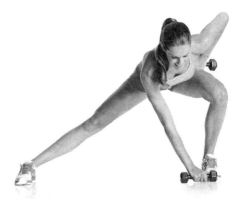

STEP-OUT BRIDGE

Lie faceup with your hands on your hips, knees bent, and feet on the floor, ankles under your knees. Lift your hips and toes and step forward with right foot [shown] and then left; step back to starting position to complete 1 rep.

TIP If this is too challenging, keep your hips on the floor.

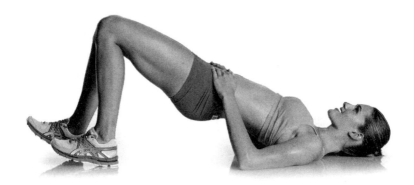

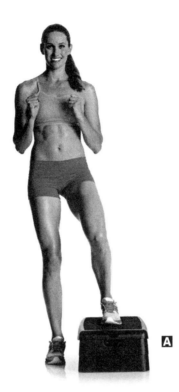

BENCH CROSS

Stand with your left foot on top of a step or bench and your right foot on the floor beside it, hands in fists in front of your shoulders **A**. Rise up as you cross your right leg behind left, then land with your right foot on the floor on the opposite side of the step **B**.
Return to starting position. Switch sides to complete the set.

TIP To increase the workload, hold a dumbbell in each hand.

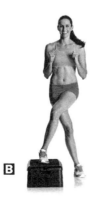

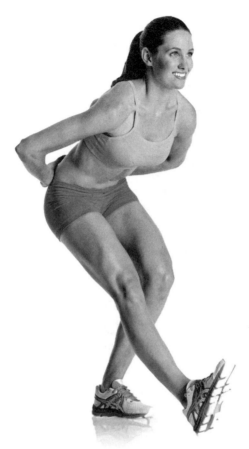

KNEE IN/OUT

Stand with feet hip width and squat.
Lean forward 45 degrees and place the
backs of your hands on your lower back.
Quickly extend your right leg straight out
in front of you [shown], return to start,
then extend right leg straight behind you.
Return to starting position to complete
1 rep. Switch sides to complete set.

TIP Imagine your hips are two headlights
that should always point straight ahead.

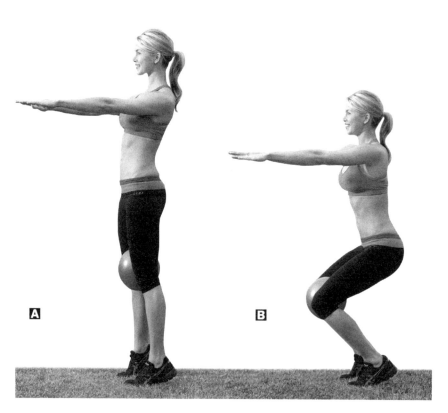

QUAD QUIVER

Stand with your feet hip-width apart and place a Pilates or playground ball between your knees. Rise up onto the balls of your feet and raise your arms to chest height in front of you, palms facing the ground **A**; squat **B**. Hold for 3 seconds, then rise up to starting position.

TIP Imagine you're about to sit down in a chair—push your hips back as you bend your knees.

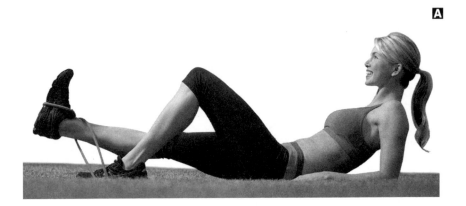

LEG LIFT

Sit with your right leg extended in front of you, foot flexed, and left knee bent, foot on the ground. Wrap a resistance tube around your right foot and place your left foot on the other end. Lean back, lowering onto your forearms, and raise your right leg until tube is taut **A**. Point your toes as you lift your right leg until your thighs are parallel **B**. Flex your foot as you lower to starting position. Switch sides to complete set.

TIP Do not lower your leg all the way back to the ground; there should always be tension in the tube.

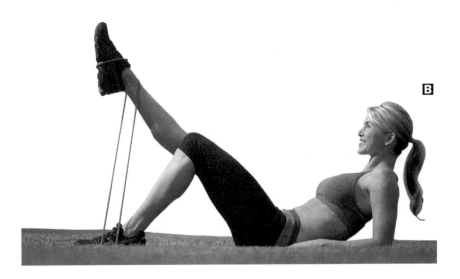

SIDE-LYING SQUEEZE

Lie on your right side with your right forearm on the ground. Place a Pilates or playground ball between your ankles and extend your legs. Squeeze the ball as you raise your legs a few inches [shown]. Lower to starting position. Switch sides to complete set.

TIP To increase the challenge on your inner thighs, squeeze the ball as hard as you can the entire time.

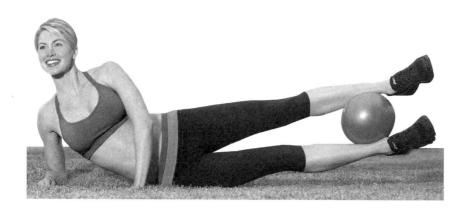

Get Even

When you do a single-leg exercise, your weaker side
can't rely on your stronger one to help it.
This results in more balanced strengthening.

CHAPTER 9

Your Bikini Body Beyond 6 Weeks

Bonus Moves to Keep You Motivated All Year Long

There tend to be two kinds of exercisers: The ones who do the same thing all the time—every day, the same routine. And the ones who like to mix it up all the time, and "just get out there." The best path: a mix of the two. It's smart to stick to a plan to maintain consistency so you can see progress. But when you do the same thing over

The Bikini Body Diet

and over, your body adapts by figuring out what it needs to do, and that's when you plateau (be it with weight or with strength gains). So for the best results, you need to mix things up. That's why the Bikini Body Diet workout works so well—you'll vary your strength and cardio workouts.

But if you're the kind of person who likes to have options, this chapter is for you. I'm including 182 more moves that will target the bikini-baring body parts of your core, legs, and butt so you can create your own workouts. There's a lot of value in doing so: A recent study at the University of South Carolina-Upstate found that when people focused on using a specific body part while executing an exercise, muscle activity in that area increased by up to 26 percent. (Researchers say it may be because the brain sends more signals to those areas, thus making more muscle fibers fire away.) So the very act of mentally targeting a certain body part actually bolsters your physical improvement in that very area.

Best of all, you can put these exercises together in a number of ways, based on the equipment you have access to, how much time you have, or what you'd like to target. Some ideas for creating your own exercise routine:

Pick four or five exercises. Do the prescribed number of reps, or duration, and run through the circuit four or five times.

In a time crunch? Pick 10 exercises and perform each for a minute with 10 seconds of rest in between.

Pick two exercises that work different body parts (say legs and core). Do them back to back, then do 2 minutes of high-intensity cardio, like jumping rope or running. Repeat.

See something you especially like? Sub it into one of the workouts in the previous chapter.

Watching your favorite show? Pick four exercises, do each for 30 seconds during the commercial breaks.

See, the point is that you can use your creativity and flexibility to create workouts that best fit into your schedule and lifestyle. For the first six weeks, I want you to follow the workouts and plan I've outlined in the previous chapters, and of course, you can continue them afterwards. But after that, you can use these moves to create a plan that will help you create your lifelong bikini body.

TARGET: Abs & Core

SIDE-LYING V-UP
Works abs

Lie on your left side with legs stacked, your left arm on the ground and right arm extended at your side; lift your legs. Roll back onto your butt and sit up as you pull your knees toward your chest and reach your right arm forward. Roll down to starting position and repeat. Switch sides after 30 second to complete set.

OUT-IN CRUNCH
Works core

Lie faceup with legs extended over your hips. Crunch up as you lower your legs out to the sides and reach your hands between them, palms pressed together. Bring your legs together again and reach hands forward on either side of thighs to complete 1 rep. Do 8 to 10 reps.

JACKKNIFE
Works core

Lie faceup with your arms overhead and legs extended toward the ground wall in front of you. Crunch up as you raise your legs 45 degrees and reach hands toward your toes. Lower to starting position. Do 8 to 10 reps.

SCISSORS
Works core

Lie faceup with your legs extended on the ground in front of you and arms at your sides, hands under your butt. Raise legs 6 to 12 inches. Then open legs as wide as your shoulders, and then cross the right leg over the left. Open legs again, and cross left over right. Continue, alternating legs for 20 seconds.

SUPERWOMAN
Works core

Lie facedown with arms overhead, palms on the ground, and legs extended, shoulder-width apart. Raise chest and legs simultaneously. Lower to starting position. Do 5 reps.

ROLL-OUT
Works abs

Kneel and place your hands, fingers clasped, on a weighted ball in front of you. Roll the ball forward until your body is aligned from head to knees, and your forearms are on the ball. Roll back to starting position. Do 12 to 15 reps.

★ CELEBRITY WORKOUT SECRET ★

A Maria Menounos Favorite!

SINKING BOAT
Works abs

Sit with knees bent and feet on the ground. Lean back until you feel your abs engage. Extend your arms at chest height in front of you, as you extend legs at diagonal in front of you. Inhale as you bring your arms out to sides, lowering your torso and legs toward the ground. Exhale as you rise up to starting position. Repeat for 1 minute.

★ CELEBRITY WORKOUT SECRET ★

A Pink Favorite!

LONG LEG ROTATION
Works core

Lie faceup with legs extended over your hips, hands behind head, and elbows pointing out to the sides. Crunch up, lifting your head and shoulders. Lower your left leg toward the floor as you rotate to the right, bringing your left elbow toward your right knee. Return to starting position; repeat on opposite side. Do 15 to 20 reps, alternating sides each rep.

PLANK JACK
Works core

Get in a modified plank position (elbows aligned under shoulders). Tighten abs so your body is straight from head to heels. Keeping your torso tight, hop your feet out wide. Hop feet back to starting position and repeat. Do 12 to 15 reps.

SEATED BICYCLE
Works abs and legs

Sit with your knees bent and feet on the ground. Lean back 45 degrees and place your hands behind your head. Extend your right leg 12 inches off the ground in front of you. Twist torso to the right as you bend your right knee, bringing your left elbow toward your right knee. Return to stating position and repeat. Do 12 to 15 reps, then switch sides to complete set.

LONG-LEVER CRUNCH
Works abs

Lie faceup with your arms extended next to your head, palms together. Place your left foot flat on the ground and extend

★ CELEBRITY WORKOUT SECRET ★

A Jordin Sparks Favorite!

MOUNTAIN CLIMBER
Works core, butt, and legs

Get in plank position, feet hip-width apart. Pull your right knee toward your chest. Extend your right leg as you pull your left knee toward your chest to complete 1 rep. Do 15 to 20 reps.

your right leg a few inches above the ground. Lift your head and shoulder blades as you raise your right leg 45 degrees so your thighs are even. Return to starting position and repeat, keeping your arms even with your ears the entire time. Do 15 to 20 reps, then switch legs to complete set.

CRAB REACH
Works abs

Sit with your hands on floor behind you, fingers pointing out and knees bent, feet about 6 inches from your butt. Lift your hips several inches, then raise your right leg and touch your left hand to your right calf. Return to starting position (hips stay up) and repeat. Do 8 to 10 reps, then switch sides to complete set. (Start with knees bent if that's easier.)

BALL SLAM
Works core, butt, and legs

Stand with your feet wider than your shoulders and place a medicine ball (preferably a no-bounce one) on the ground in front of you. Squat low and pick up the ball. Rise up, raise ball overhead, and immediately slam it down on the ground in front of you; repeat. Do 20 to 25 reps.

PLANK TO UPWARD-FACING DOG
Works core

Get in plank position with your body aligned from shoulders to heels. Bend your elbows straight back behind you, lowering your chest toward the ground; lift your chest, arch your back, and look up. Reverse motion to return to the starting position. Do 12 to 15 reps.

ROLL DOWN
Works core

Sit up tall with your knees bent and feet on the floor in front of you, hip-width apart. Extend your arms at shoulder height in front of you, palms pressed together. Pull abs in and roll back as you bring arms overhead, stopping just before your shoulders hit the floor. Immediately roll up to the starting position. Do 12 to 15 reps.

SEESAW CRUNCH
Works abs

Sit with your knees bent and hands on the floor behind you, fingers facing forward. Raise legs so your shins are parallel to floor, and lean back, elbows slightly bent, until you feel your abs engage.

★ CELEBRITY WORKOUT SECRET ★

A Nicole Scherzinger Favorite!

REVERSE CHOP
Works core

Hold a weighted ball with both hands in front of hips, and stand with feet wider than your shoulders, knees slightly bent. Rotate shoulders to the left, brining the ball outside left hip. Twist torso to right as you raise ball up at diagonal to right. Return to starting position. Switch sides to complete set. Do 12 to 15 reps.

Extend legs straight out in front of you as you lean back farther. Return to starting position. Do 12 to 15 reps.

STANDING CRUNCH TO SQUAT
Works abs, butt, and legs

Stand with feet slightly wider than your shoulders, hands behind your head, elbows out to your sides. Bend from the hips to the right as you bring your right knee toward your elbow. Return to starting position, then immediately repeat with left knee and elbow. Return to the starting position, then squat. Repeat the entire sequence at a fast pace. Do 12 to 15 reps.

CROSS-LEG LIFT
Works abs

Lie faceup with legs extended over hips and arms at your sides, palms on the ground. Bend your right knee, crossing your right foot over your left thigh. Keeping the left leg straight, use your abs to lift your hips off the ground. Lower your hips, then take legs down to 45 degrees off the ground. Raise legs back up and repeat entire move. Switch legs (crossing left leg over right) halfway through the set. Do 12 to 15 reps on each side.

★ CELEBRITY WORKOUT SECRET ★

A Marisa Miller Favorite!

BURPEE
Works entire body

Stand with feet shoulder-width apart, then squat and put your hands on the floor in front of feet. Hop feet back, then forward again; jump up, raising hands overhead. Add a pushup while you're in plank pose for more of a challenge. Do 12 to 15 reps.

V-UP TUCK AND PIKE
Works abs

Lie faceup with your legs extended on the floor in front of you and hands behind head; lift your legs 45 degrees. Bend knees in toward your chest as you sit up, wrapping your hands around your legs. Return to starting position. Do 15 reps. Next, keep legs extended and raise them higher as you sit up, reaching hands toward your feet. Hold for 1 count, then return to start. Do 5 reps.

TARGET: Legs & Butt

WONDER WOMAN
Works core, butt, and legs

Stand with feet a stride's length apart, left in front of right, and hands in fists in front of your shoulders. Bend your knees until your left thigh is parallel to the ground. Rise up as you bend forward from the hips, raising your right leg to hip height behind you and extending arms at your sides. Return to starting position. Switch legs after 30 seconds.

BOOTY BOOSTER
Works butt and legs

Lie faceup, knees bent and feet on the ground. Extend arms at your sides and raise left leg, thighs parallel. Lift hips. Keeping left leg raised, lower your body to starting position. Switch legs after 30 seconds.

KNEELING LEG LIFT
Works core and outer thighs

Get in a side plank position on your left side, and lower your left knee to the ground; place your right hand behind your head. Lift right leg to hip height, then lower back to starting position. Switch sides after 30 seconds.

★ CELEBRITY WORKOUT SECRET ★

An Alison Sweeney Favorite!

DEADLIFT
Works core, butt, and legs

Stand holding dumbbells or a light bar with your feet shoulder-width apart, hands slightly wider than your hips and palms facing your body. Keep a straight lower back as you bend your knees, lowering the bar toward to the floor. Rise up to starting position. Do 8 to 10 reps.

HOT FEET
Works core, butt, and legs

Stand with feet hip-width apart, then step out with your right foot, bring your left foot next to it, step out again with your right foot (step-together-step), and bring your left knee and right elbow together. Repeat back and forth as fast as possible 10 times (5 times in each direction). Then stand with feet wider than your shoulders, lower into a squat and bring your hands together in front of you, elbows bent. Alternate quickly lifting your left foot and then right a few inches. After 15 seconds, bring feet in close and then continue, taking your feet wide again after another 15 seconds. Repeat for 30 more seconds.

SINGLE-LEG KICK
Works butt

Lie facedown with elbows bent at your sides, palms on the mat. Press palms down and lift your chest. Keeping your upper body raised, bend and lift your left knee and pulse your left foot toward your butt twice. Extend your left leg and repeat pulses with right foot to complete 1 rep. Do 20 total reps.

HEEL-TOE TAP
Works butt

Get on all fours, shoulders over wrists and hips over knees, and extend your right leg at hip height beside you, placing your foot on a chair. Rotate right leg back so your heel is on the seat and toes point toward the ceiling. Quickly rotate your right leg forward, placing toes on the chair. Continue for 30 seconds, then switch sides to complete set.

ULTIMATE BUTT BURNER
Works butt and legs

Get on all fours and position a weighted ball behind your left knee, foot flexed; bend your knee so the ball is secure. Raise your leg straight up behind you, then lower. Next, raise your leg out to the left so thigh is parallel to the ground, then lower. Finally, lift left leg and cross it over your right behind you, to complete 1 rep. Do 12 to 15 reps, then switch sides to complete set.

PLYO SPLIT SQUAT
Works butt

Stand with the ball of your left foot on a step or bench behind you. Squat low, placing your hands on the floor on either side of your right foot. Jump up and land in the starting position. Do 10 reps, then switch legs to complete set.

BALL SQUAT
Works butt and legs

Stand with a stability ball between your back and a wall, walk your feet forward until they're slightly in front of your hips, and place your hands on your thighs. Squat until your thighs are parallel to the floor. Rise up onto balls of your feet as you reach your arms overhead. Return to starting position and do 12 reps.

ROLLING BRIDGE
Works abs, butt, and legs

Lie faceup, squeezing a stability ball between your lower legs. Raise your hips up and back. Roll the ball to the left, lowering left leg toward the ground. Return to the starting position and repeat, rolling to the right. Continue alternating sides for 30 seconds.

BALANCE SQUAT
Works core, butt, and legs

Stand with feet shoulder-width apart on the flat side of a Bosu (or use the round side if that's more comfortable for you) and hold a dumbbell in each hand at your sides. Squat as low as you can, maintaining your balance and keeping your knees aligned with your thighs, then rise up and repeat. Do 12 to 15 reps.

★ CELEBRITY WORKOUT SECRET ★

A Kate Walsh Favorite!

GLUTE SWEEP
Works butt

Stand facing a wall with feet wide, toes turned out, and arms extended at chest height in front of you, palms pressed against wall. Bend your knees, then rise up on your right leg as you keep your left leg bent and press it up behind you. Return to starting position. Do 12 to 15 reps; repeat on opposite side to complete set.

BALL SKATE
Works abs, butt, and legs

Stand holding a stability ball in front of you with your arms extended. Hop to the left, extending your right leg behind your left as you reach the ball toward your right foot. Hop to the right, crossing your left leg behind you and swinging the ball toward your left foot. Continue hopping from side to side, doing 12 reps each way.

CURTSY RAISE
Works butt

Stand on bottom steps, facing upstairs, feet together and hands on hips. Step back and to the left with your right foot and bend your knees. Rise up as you extend your right leg out to the side, foot flexed. Return to the starting position. Switch sides after 30 seconds.

LUNGE HOP
Works butt and legs

Stand with feet hip-width apart, arms bent at your sides and hands in fists. Lunge back with your right leg, bending both knees 90 degrees, your right arm forward and left arm back (as if you're running). Rise up onto your left leg and jump, bringing your right knee to hip height in front of you as you switch arms. Land and immediately step back to starting position. Do 15 to 20 reps, then switch sides to complete set.

QUAD QUIVER
Works core, butt, and legs

Stand with feet hip-width apart and place a Pilates ball between your knees. Rise up onto the balls of your feet and raise arms to chest height in front of you, palms facing ground; squat. Hold for 3 seconds, then rise up to starting position. Do 15 to 20 reps.

TRIPOD KICK
Works core and butt

Get on all fours with forearms and palms on the ground and a loop resistance band around your feet; lift your right foot off the ground. Extend your right leg to hip height behind you, then return to starting position. Next extend your right leg on the ground behind you, then raise it as high as you can without arching your back. Lower leg to starting position. Do 15 to 20 reps. Repeat entire series on opposite side to complete set.

WOBBLY TOUCHDOWN
Works core, butt, and legs

Stand with your right foot on a pillow and left knee raised to hip height in front of you. Extend your arms at shoulder height out to the side, palms facing floor. Bend your right knee, hinge forward from your hips, and reach your left hand toward floor as you extend left leg to hip height behind you. Rise up to the starting position. Switch sides after 30 seconds.

PENDULUM
Works abs and butt

Stand with feet shoulder-width apart and bend over from your hips, keeping your back as flat as possible. Place hands on a weighted

★ CELEBRITY WORKOUT SECRET ★

A Kourtney Kardashian Favorite!

LOW WALKING
Works butt and legs

Stand with feet hip-width apart and extend arms in front of you, hands clasped. Squat low and walk forward 20 steps, then backward 20 steps.

★ CELEBRITY WORKOUT SECRET ★

A Jenny McCarthy Favorite!

BOOTY LIFT
Works butt

Get on all fours with a dumbbell clasped behind your right knee, and pull abs in so your back is flat. Raise right knee to hip height behind you, foot flexed, and lower to starting position. Do 12 to 15 reps, then hold right knee up at hip height behind you for 10 seconds. Switch sides to complete set.

---

ball on the floor in front of your feet (or rest ball on a low step); hands should be aligned under your chin. Keeping hands flat on the ball, raise your left leg out to the side to hip height; hold for 2 counts, then switch sides to complete 1 rep. Do 12 to 15 reps.

SLIDING LUNGE
Works core, butt, and legs

Stand with your right foot on a towel and hands on your hips. Slide your right foot back as you bend your knees, lowering into a lunge. Return to starting position. Switch sides after 30 seconds.

KNEELING ARABESQUE
Works butt and legs

Get on all fours, wrists aligned under shoulders and knees under hips. Extend your left leg behind you, foot on the floor and toes pointed. Lift your leg behind you, then lower to starting position. Do 12 to 15 reps, then switch sides to complete set.

BRIDGE
Works core, butt, and legs

Place a foam roller horizontally against a wall, and lie faceup in front of it with knees bent, feet hip-width apart on the roller and heels on the floor. Place your hands behind your head, elbows out to the sides. Press your hips up until body forms a line from knees to shoulders. Lower to starting position. Do 15 to 20 reps.

BALL SQUEEZE
Works quads and inner thighs

Sit on the edge of a bench with your legs extended in front of you, knees slightly bent. Place a weighted ball between your knees and lift your toes so your heels are down and feet are parallel. Squeeze your legs together and straighten your knees without hyperextending them; heels should stay on the ground. Hold for 3 counts, then release and repeat. Do 15 to 20 reps.

PLIÉ SQUAT
Works butt and legs

Stand with feet wide, toes turned out; hold a dumbbell in each hand in front of your hips, palms facing body. Rise onto the balls of your feet (heels up) and lower into a squat. Straighten legs (keeping heels lifted) and repeat. Do 10 reps.

PISTOL SQUAT
Works butt and legs

Stand with feet slightly wider than your shoulders and extend both arms at shoulder height in front of you; bend your right knee to lift your leg off the ground. Extend your right leg at hip height in front of you, foot flexed. Bend your left knee to descend, then rise up to starting position. Do 12 reps, then switch sides to complete set.

POWER HOP
Works core, butt, and legs

Stand with your left knee bent and hands in fists as your sides. Hop to the left. Then bend your right knee, reaching your left hand toward the ground as you extend your right arm behind you.

Rise up to starting position and repeat. Continues for 30 seconds, then switch sides to complete set.

HARDCORE SQUAT
Works core, butt, and legs

Stand with feet shoulder-width apart, hands behind your ears, and squat. Rise up as you raise your right knee to hip height in front of you and rotate shoulders to right. Twist back to center as you jump up and kick your left foot forward. Return to starting position; repeat on opposite side to complete 1 rep. Do 10 reps.

SCOOTER
Works core, butt, and legs

Stand with the top of your right foot on a stability ball and raise arms to chest height in front of you, palms facing the ground. Roll ball back as you squat on your left leg. Rise to starting position and repeat. Do 10 reps, then switch sides to complete set.

★ CELEBRITY WORKOUT SECRET ★

A Brooke Burke Favorite!

REVERSE LUNGE SWEEP
Works core, butt, and legs

Stand with feet hip-width apart and hands in fists in front of chin, palms facing each other. Lunge back with your left leg. Rise up, shifting weight to your right leg as you sweep your left leg straight out to the side and then raise it high in front of you; touch your left foot with your right hand as you extend your left arm behind you. Lunge back again with the left leg and repeat. Do 12 reps, then switch sides to complete the set.

ROUNDHOUSE KICK
Works core, butt, and legs

Hold a light bar or broomstick with your right hand in front of your chest, left hand open and over left shoulder, and stand with feet together. Inhale as you raise your right knee to hip height out to the side, foot flexed, and lean torso to the left, then exhale as you extend your right leg. Return to the starting position and immediately repeat. Do 10 reps, then switch legs to complete set.

OFFSET BRIDGE
Works core, butt, and legs

Lie faceup with right knee bent, foot on the ground, and left leg extended over your hips. Extend arms at your sides, palms on the ground. Push through your right heel as you lift your hips until your body is aligned from your shoulders to right knee. Lower your hips until they nearly touch the ground, then repeat. Do 10 reps, then switch sides to complete set.

SIDE RUNNING
Works butt, and inner and outer thighs

Run to the side for 30 seconds. Step out to the left with your left foot, then bring your right foot in next to it as you step out again with your left foot (don't cross legs in front of each other).

★ CELEBRITY WORKOUT SECRET ★

A Vanessa Hudgens Favorite!

BOX JUMP
Works butt and legs

Stand facing box or step, feet shoulder-width apart and arms extended at your sides. Squat, then jump onto the plyo box, using your arms to propel you. Step down to return to starting position and repeat. Do 15 to 20 reps.

★ CELEBRITY WORKOUT SECRET ★

A Jennifer Love Hewitt Favorite!

DROP DOWN
Works butt and legs

Stand with feet wide and parallel. Bend forward from your hips and extend your arms straight down from your shoulders until fingertips touch the floor; look straight ahead. Rotate toes out as you squat low. Return to the starting position. Continue for 45 seconds.

Alternate between taking smaller strides—maybe 18 inches wide— and wider strides (2 feet or more). Continue for 30 seconds, then switch directions and repeat. Do 4 runs to each side.

OVER-THE-TOP SHUFFLE
Works butt and legs

Stand with your right side next to an adjustable step (or a curb). Place right foot on the center of the step and bring left foot out so feet are wide, bend elbows at your sides, and squat slightly. (If you're using a curb, jump on and off with both feet.) Push off your right foot and hop over to the right side of the step, landing with your right foot on the ground and left foot on the step. Repeat, jumping from side to side, for 2 minutes. (If you're using a curb, switch sides after 1 minute.)

DIAGONAL SWING
Works core, butt, and legs

Stand with feet together, knees slightly bent. Bend forward from your hips, crossing arms overhead, hands in fists. Raise torso 45 degrees as you lift your left heel and rotate your shoulders

to the left, extending your right arm in front of you and left arm
behind you. Return to starting position; repeat, rotating to the
right. Continue at a quick pace, alternating sides for 2 minutes.

KNEE-IN/OUT
Works core, butt, and legs

Stand with feet hip-width apart and squat. Lean forward
45 degrees and place the backs of your hands on your lower
back. Quickly extend right leg straight back behind you, return
to starting position, then extend right leg straight out in front
of you and back to starting position to complete 1 rep. Do
10 reps. Switch sides to complete set.

LEG RAISE AND CIRCLE
Works outer thighs and legs

Stand with hands on hips. Shift your weight to your left leg and lift
your right leg out to the side, then lower it until it nearly touches
the floor. Do 20 reps. Next, raise your right leg out to the side and
circle it forward 10 times and back 10 times (circles should be about
6 inches in diameter). Switch sides to complete the set.

CLOCK LUNGE
Works butt and legs

Stand with feet hip-width apart. Lunge forward with your right
foot, step back to starting position, and then lunge back with your
right foot. Return to starting position, then lunge to the right with
your right foot. Step back to starting position. Repeat on opposite
side to complete set. Do 10 reps with each leg.

DOUBLE LEG LIFT
Works inner and outer thighs

Lie on your right side with a medicine ball between your ankles.
Rest your head on your right arm and place your left hand on

floor in front of you for balance. Keeping legs straight, and hips and shoulders squared forward, lift both legs several inches. Lower almost all the way to the floor and repeat. Switch sides after 30 seconds.

180 PLYO
Works butt and legs

Stand with feet wide, toes turned out. Squat, then jump up and turn 180 degrees. When you land, lower into a deep squat. Jump back to starting position and repeat to other side. Do 10 jumps each direction.

BRIDGE WALK
Works butt and legs

Lie faceup, with feet flat on a low bench or step, arms at sides. Lift hips 5 inches, then lift left foot then right foot a few inches off step. Try to "walk" as quickly as possible for 60 seconds, holding up hips.

SIDE WALL SLIDE
Works core, butt, and legs

Place a stability ball against a wall and lean your left side against it, feet together and weight on right the leg. Raise left arm to chest

★ CELEBRITY WORKOUT SECRET ★

An Elisha Cuthbert Favorite!

SQUAT RAISE
Works butt and legs

Stand with feet slightly wider than your shoulders and arms extended at sides. Squat as you raise your arms to chest height in front of you, palms facing floor. Lower your arms to your sides as your rise up and lift your left knee to hip height in front of you. Repeat, this time raising right knee. Continue at a quick pace, alternating knees. Do 15 to 20 reps on each leg.

height in front of you, palm facing the ground, and place right hand on hip. Step your left foot at a diagonal behind you as you bend your right knee. Press against the ball as you return to starting position. Do 12 to 15 reps. Switch sides to complete set.

CLAMSHELL
Works butt and outer thighs

Tie a resistance band around your thighs, just above your knees, and lie on your left side with your knees bent and legs stacked, left arm extended and right hand on floor in front of chest. Keeping feet together, lift your right leg. Return to starting position. Do 12 reps, then switch sides to complete side.

CRISSCROSS JUMPING JACKS
Works butt and legs

Stand with feet together, arms at your sides, and jump feet wide as you raise your arms out to shoulder height. Lower into a squat, then jump back to starting position, crossing your left foot behind right and lowering your arms to sides; land with knees bent.

★ CELEBRITY WORKOUT SECRET ★

A Molly Sims Favorite!

SIDE-LYING KNEE-IN
Works butt and outer thighs

Lie on left side with left elbow bent, weight on forearm, and right hand on mat in front of you. Bend your knees, place your right foot behind your left ankle, and raise your left foot, toes pointed. Lift right knee, then extend your right leg out at a diagonal to the side. Bend right knee and repeat, keeping left calf raised. Return to starting position. Do 12 reps each side.

Jump feet wide again, then switch legs to complete 1 rep.
Do 15 to 20 reps.

EYE-HIGH KICK
Works core and legs

Stand with feet together, knees slightly bent, and place your
hands on your hips with fingers pointing toward the floor.
Jump up as you kick your left leg high, toes pointed. Return
to starting position and immediately repeat on opposite side
to complete 1 rep. Do 8 reps.

LUNGE AND KICK
Works core, butt, and legs

Stand with elbows at chest height out to sides, hands stacked
and palms facing floor. Lunge back with your left foot as you
rotate your shoulders to the left. Rise up as you kick your left
leg in front of you and extend your right arm forward and
left arm back. Step back to starting position Continue for
1 minute, then repeat on opposite side.

The Upper-Body-Sculpting Workout

There's a lot that goes into having your best bikini body, but it's not
always about what's going on below the waist. Having sexy shoulders is a
symbol of strength and confidence. These ballet-inspired moves will give
you a strong and sleek upper body. (Bonus: because you'll be standing
in traditional ballet postures, your legs and butt will get a workout too!)
Do 1 set of 12 reps of each exercise without resting between moves.
Repeat the circuit once or twice. Use light dumbbells (3 to 5 pounds).

PLIÉ PUNCH
Works shoulders, chest, back, legs, and butt

Stand in plié position (feet wide, toes turned out, and knees bent) and squat. Hold weights in front of your shoulders, elbows out to your sides and palms facing floor. Punch forward with your left arm. Bend your left elbow to return to starting position; repeat on opposite side to complete 1 rep.

BALLET CURL
Works biceps

Stand in first position (heels together, toes out), and hold weights at shoulder height out to sides, palms facing ceiling. Bend your left elbow, bringing your hand toward your head. Return to starting position; repeat with right arm to complete 1 rep.

BALANCE PULSE
Works triceps and core

Stand with feet together and hold a weight in each hand at sides, palms facing behind you. Bend forward from your hips

★ CELEBRITY WORKOUT SECRET ★

A Cindy Crawford Favorite!

TOE BRIDGE
Works core, butt, and legs

Lie faceup with knees bent and the balls of your feet on the floor, heels close to your butt. Extend arms at your sides, palms on the floor. Lift your hips until your body is aligned from knees to shoulders. Lower to starting position and repeat, keeping your heels raised the entire time.

and bend your right knee, shifting weight to your left leg. Raise arms behind you; lower arms to starting position. Switch legs halfway through set.

PLIÉ FLY
Works chest, butt, and legs

Stand in plié position and hold a weight in each hand, elbows bent 90 degrees and raised to shoulder height and palms facing forward. Bring hands toward each other in front of you, palms facing your face. Return to starting position.

WINDSHIELD WIPER
Works triceps, butt, and legs

Stand in plié position and bend forward slightly from the hips. Hold weights in front of your chest, turning them perpendicular to the floor, with palms facing body. Lower weights in front of you, and then raise them out to sides, so palms face behind you. Return to starting position.

WINDMILL
Works shoulders, back, butt, and legs

Stand in plié position, squat deep, and bend forward slightly from hips. Hold weights between your legs, palms facing each other and elbows slightly bent. Rise up as you rotate your right shoulder back and raise your right arm straight up. Return to starting position; repeat on opposite side to complete 1 rep.

CHAPTER 10

The Summer Body Workout Guide

Fun On-the-Go Sweat Sessions

Say the word *summer* and you're likely to think of bikinis (natch) and beaches, lemonade and lounging, hammocks and hotels. And while it's prime vacation time, I also know that lots of people take that time off from diets and exercise. There's nothing wrong with the occasional break, of course, and I don't want you to spend all your time off obsessing about when and how you're going to work out. But I also know that vacations, holidays, or business travel can be the veritable safety pin to the balloon of an exercise program—immediately destroying it.

To that end, I want to give you even more options for working out while you're on the road. Some of these are summer-friendly workouts that you can use when you're on the beach or outdoors, but many of them are ones you can do no matter where you are and no matter what time of year. They are fast, don't require a lot of equipment, and are all about helping you get your best bikini body.

Of course, you can always use the Bikini Body Diet workouts in the previous chapters, and you can mix and match moves and plans to fit your schedule, if you like. But I wanted to give you even more options, so you can construct workouts no matter your goals, your environment, and how you feel on a particular day.

Here, you'll find some of my favorite fast workouts that will challenge your body in a short amount of time. That way, you can always maximize your off time—and still feel *on*.

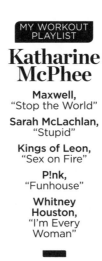

MY WORKOUT PLAYLIST

Katharine McPhee

Maxwell,
"Stop the World"

Sarah McLachlan,
"Stupid"

Kings of Leon,
"Sex on Fire"

P!nk,
"Funhouse"

Whitney Houston,
"I'm Every Woman"

The Mariah Carey Water Workout

A great, low-impact (and sexy) way to work all of your muscles: Hit the pool. That's how Mariah Carey slimmed down after having twins. (Swimming is her favorite form of exercise.) After you swim laps, do five sets of these moves, designed by Mariah, to boost the sculpting benefits of your water workout even more.

STATIONARY KICK

Stand in the shallow end and hold the edge of the pool with hands shoulder-width apart, elbows bent. Extend legs, and keeping feet together, kick hard, starting the movement in your hips. Continue for 30 seconds to complete set.

BUTTERFLY HUG

Stand in chest-level water with arms extended at shoulder height out to sides, palms facing down. Jump, bringing your knees toward your chest, as you press palms together in front of you. Return to starting position. Do 5 reps to complete set.

BUTTERFLY BEAT

Stand with feet together and arms extended at sides. Keeping arms underwater, clap hands together in front of you, then behind you. Continue, alternating claps forward and back, for 30 seconds to complete set.

MERMAID MOMENT

Place a pool noodle under your chest, so your shoulders are out of the water; extend legs behind you, feet together. Bend your knees, then extend legs, propelling yourself across the pool. Continue for 30 seconds to complete set.

The Britney Spears Yoga Workout

When you want to strengthen your entire body—while getting a soothing stretch—yoga can't be beat. And because it requires no equipment, this ancient practice is ideal for hotel rooms. During yoga, you engage your entire core and nearly every other muscle group. Plus, holding positions helps increase your flexibility and calm your mind. One of our *Shape* cover girls, Britney Spears, knows a thing or two about keeping her body fit, and she loves to do the following yoga workout. Perform each pose in order. Repeat the series up to three times. Don't worry if you can't do the moves perfectly at first; keep at it and you'll gradually feel the difference as your body becomes stronger and more limber.

BOAT
Works core and legs

Sit up tall with knees bent and arms extended at chest height in front of you. Sit back until you feel your abs engage, then slowly lift your feet until shins are parallel to the floor. (Advanced yogis can extend legs at a 45-degree angle.) Hold for 3 deep breaths—inhale and exhale through your nose, taking at least 5 counts for each—then lower your feet to the floor. Rest for 30 seconds, Repeat twice more.

CRESCENT LUNGE
Strengthens butt and legs; stretches hip flexors

Stand with feet together and arms extended at sides, palms facing thighs. Take a big step forward with your left leg and bend your left knee (until thigh is parallel to the floor, if you can); keep right leg extended and heel lifted. Extend arms overhead and press palms together. Hold for 5 to 10 breaths and then lower your arms. Then step your right foot forward (so it comes next to the left) and repeat on the opposite side.

WARRIOR 2

Strengthens shoulders and legs; stretches chest and legs

Stand with feet together, arms extended at sides. Take a step forward with your left leg; turn your right foot out so it's even with left heel. Bend your left knee (until thigh is parallel to the floor, if you can), raise arms to shoulder height to the sides, and look over left fingertips. Hold for 5 breaths, then step your right foot forward (next to the left), and repeat on the opposite side.

BOW

Strengthens back; stretches abs, chest, shoulders, and legs

Lie facedown with legs hip-width part and arms extended at sides. Inhale and bend your knees as you reach your hands behind you, grasping the outsides of your ankles. Exhale and press your ankles against your hands as you lift your thighs. Hold for 5 breaths, then return to starting position.

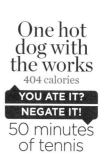

One hot dog with the works
404 calories

**YOU ATE IT?
NEGATE IT!**

50 minutes of tennis

CAMEL

Strengthens arms and shoulders; stretches shoulders, chest, abs, and legs

Kneel with legs hip-width apart, then arch back and reach for your right heel with your right hand, then your left heel with your left hand. Lift chest, press hips forward, and drop head back. Hold for 5 to 10 breaths. Reverse the motion to come out of the pose.

The Dance It Off Workout

There's no question that Beyoncé has one of the most beautiful bodies in the world. And diet has a lot to do with it: The star keeps a very Bikini Body Diet–like eating plan. For breakfast, she eats scrambled egg whites, a vegetable smoothie, or whole-grain cereal with low-fat milk. And for lunch and dinner, she eats fish and veggies (and she also allows herself one cheat meal on Sundays). To help keep her body lean and fit, it's all about the moves. The dance moves. She credits dancing with giving her a strong and sexy body. While you can achieve the same effects with many of the workouts you'll find in this book, there's also nothing wrong with getting your groove on. Dancing can burn up to 450 calories an hour, and a study in the *Journal of Sports Science & Medicine* found that Zumba in particular buns about 570 calories an hour. It doesn't matter where you dance—in a class, in a club, or in your jammies before bed!

To add some more lower-body sculpting to your dance workout, try this chair-based plan from Miami-based Zumba specialist Melissa Chiz. Do 1 set of 12 reps of each move in order, then repeat the series twice more. (To increase the calorie burn, dance for 30 seconds between each exercise.)

CROSSOVER
Works inner and outer thighs

Sit on the edge of a chair's seat with feet shoulder-width apart on the floor and grasp sides of the chair with your hands. Lift your right leg and bring it toward your left, crossing your right ankle over your left. Quickly return to the starting position and repeat. Switch sides to complete set.

SIDE-STEP LUNGE
Works butt and legs

Stand behind the chair and grasp the top with hands shoulder-width apart. Take a big step to the right with your right foot and lower into a lunge. Hop or step back to starting position and repeat on left side to complete 1 rep.

REAR RAISE
Works butt and legs

Stand facing one side of the chair with feet together. Bend forward from your hips and hold the seat edge with one hand, grasping the chair back with the other hand. Bend your knees slightly and raise your right heel off the floor. Continue lifting right leg to hip height behind you, foot flexed. Lower leg to starting position and repeat. Switch legs to complete set.

SEATED BICYCLE
Works core and legs

Sit on the edge of the seat with feet hip-width apart on the floor, knees aligned over ankles; place hands behind head. Raise your left knee toward your chest as you rotate your shoulders to the left. Return to starting position and repeat on right side to complete 1 rep.

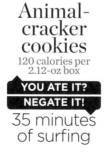

Animal-cracker cookies
120 calories per 2.12-oz box

YOU ATE IT?
NEGATE IT!
35 minutes of surfing

The Jillian Michaels 10-Minute Workout

Jillian Michaels has visited the homes of millions of Americans, as she helps contestants on *The Biggest Loser* shed pounds. Her moves and her methods work. Below is a five-exercise version of her total-body workout system called BodyShred. Do each move for 30 to 60 seconds in order. Repeat twice, taking up to a minute between circuits to catch your breath. You'll need a pair of 5- to 8-pound dumbbells.

BEAR
Works shoulders, chest, triceps, abs, and legs

Get on all fours, wrists under shoulders and knees under your hips. Curl your toes under and lift your knees off the floor. Jump your feet forward as you reach your left arm overhead and extend your right leg straight out in front of you so weight is on right hand and left foot. Reverse motion to return to starting position, and repeat on opposite side. Continue, alternating sides.

PUSH AND PRAY
Works shoulders, triceps, and legs

Get in plank position and bend elbows, lowering chest toward the floor. Push up explosively as you raise your right arm and right leg and rotate your body back, placing your right foot on the floor next to your left knee and extending your right arm toward the ceiling. Reverse motion to return to starting position. Switch direction halfway through set.

SUMO DRAGON
Works shoulders, core, butt, and legs

Stand with feet staggered and a stride's length apart, left in front of right and turned out. Hold a dumbbell in each hand overhead (at a slight angle to the left) and bend your left knee. Bend your elbows, bringing your forearms near your ears, and move the weights in a circular motion behind your head to the right as you step your right foot at a diagonal behind the left and squat as you extend your arms to the left. Reverse the motion to return to starting position. Switch sides (move in opposite direction) halfway through set.

FIGURE-4 CURL
Works biceps, butt, and legs

Stand with feet hip-width apart, holding a dumbbell in each hand with arms extended at sides and palms facing away from you. Shift weight to left foot and cross your right ankle over your left thigh. Squat as you curl weights toward your shoulders. Rise up as you extend arms to return to starting position. Switch legs halfway through set.

SIDE KICK ROLL
Works shoulders, abs, and inner and outer thighs

Get in side plank position on your left side with left forearm on the floor, elbow aligned under shoulder and knees bent. Bend your right elbow at shoulder height out to the side, hand in fist, and pull your right knee toward it. Then raise your hips as you extend your right leg and right arm at a diagonal out to the side. Return to starting position and roll to the right, landing in a side plank on your right side. Repeat. Continue, alternating sides. (If this is too tough, skip the roll and just do the kicks, switching sides halfway through the set.)

Chocolate-coated candies
240 calories per 1.69-oz bag

YOU ATE IT?
NEGATE IT!
60 minutes of walking

The Surfer Girl Workout

Surfing will net you a hot body, but learning how to do it can be intimidating. The ride seems cool enough, but that whole pop-up while you're in the mouth of a wave can take some doing. A lesson will teach you good technique, and we can help get your body ready. This yoga-inspired total-body workout will help prepare you to battle the swells—or at least look like you could. The exercises mimic actions you perform on a board, like paddling and popping up—so they strengthen all the muscles you'll use in the water. Do each pose in order; rest for 15 to 30 seconds between sets.

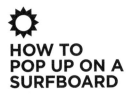

HOW TO POP UP ON A SURFBOARD

✸ Practice on land: Lie facedown on the board on land, hands under ribs, legs extended. Push your chest up, then bring one foot forward and raise your torso.

✸ When you're ready to dive in, keep your eyes on the ocean to catch a good wave.

✸ When a good wave is coming, start paddling. When you feel the wave under the board, pop up (like you did on land) with your feet wide and staggered. Bend your knees and raise your arms out to the sides for balance.

CAT/COW
Works core

Get on all fours, wrists under shoulders and knees under hips, with tops of your feet on the ground. Inhale, then exhale as you round your back, pulling abs in and drawing chin to chest. Inhale as you arch your back and look forward. Return to the starting position. Continue for 10 breaths.

WATER WARRIOR
Works core, butt, and legs

Stand with feet hip-width apart and arms extended at shoulder height in front of you, palms facing each other. Step right foot back and bend your knees, lowering into a lunge; inhale. Exhale as you rise up, drawing your right knee toward your chest and hands toward your waist. Inhale,

200

then exhale as you extend your right leg to hip height behind you, hinging forward from your hips and extending arms behind you. Hold for 5 breaths. Reverse motion to return to the starting position. Do 5 reps, then switch sides to complete set. Do 3 sets.

JUMP-SWITCH LUNGE
Works chest, shoulders, abs, butt, and legs

Get in plank position with feet hip-width apart and wrists under your shoulders. Step right foot forward between your hands. Inhale and, keeping palms or fingertips on the ground, extend your right leg back as you jump your left foot forward. Exhale, then switch, extending left leg as you jump your right foot forward. Do 3 sets of 10 reps.

DUCK DIVE
Works chest, shoulders, arms, butt, and legs

Get in plank position, then push hips up so your body forms an inverted V. Inhale as you lift your left leg high behind you. Exhale as you bend your elbows out to the sides and lower your chest toward the ground. Inhale as you bring your chest forward toward your hands and extend your arms, keeping your left leg raised the entire time. Reverse motion to return to the starting position. Do 5 reps; switch sides to complete set. Do 3 sets.

SINGLE-LEG EXTENSION
Works core, butt, and legs

Stand with feet hip-width apart, arms at sides. Inhale as you shift weight onto your left foot and lift your right knee toward your chest, clasping hands behind your thigh. Exhale as you extend your right leg to hip height or higher in front of you. Inhale as you bend your right knee to return to starting position. Do 5 reps, then release arms and keep your right leg extended for 30 seconds, slowly inhaling and exhaling through your nose. Switch sides to complete set. Do 1 set.

PADDLER'S POSE
Works back, butt, and hamstrings

Lie facedown with legs extended hip-width apart behind you and arms extended overhead, palms on the ground. Inhale as you lift your arms, chest, and legs. Exhale as you move your arms in an arc out to your sides until they're extended behind you, palms facing each other. Reverse motion to return to starting position. Do 10 reps, keeping arms, chest, and legs raised the entire time. Do 3 sets.

POP-UP VINYASA
Works chest, back, butt, and legs

Lie facedown with legs extended behind you and toes tucked; place hands under your shoulders and bend elbows. Inhale as you straighten your arms, lift your chest, and look up. Exhale as you jump your feet forward, landing with your left foot between your hands and right foot behind it, both feet angled slightly toward your right hand. Inhale, then exhale as you rise up (keep knees slightly bent), lifting arms out to your sides as if you were balancing on a surfboard. Reverse motion to return to starting position. Do 10 reps, then switch sides to complete set. Do 3 sets.

TORSO TWIST
Works abs

Lie faceup with knees bent over your hips, shins parallel to the ground and arms extended at shoulder height out to the sides, palms on the ground. Inhale, then exhale as you lower your knees to the right until they almost touch the ground. Inhale as you bring knees through center, and exhale as you lower them to the left side. Return to starting position to complete 1 rep. Do 3 sets of 5 reps.

The Summer Sand Workout

Fine-tune your whole body with a routine that challenges every muscle. You can do it on land if you like, but for more of a challenge, try it on the beach. Sand is unstable, so moving on it forces all the stabilizing muscles in your body—including those in your core—to work hard to keep you balanced. Do one set of each move in order without resting. Repeat the series twice. If you don't have gear, you can do the exercises without it, or sub in water bottles for dumbbells!

WALKOUT
Works core

Stand with feet hip-width apart, bend over from your hips, and place palms or fingertips on the ground. Keeping feet in place, walk hands forward, until you're in plank position, hands aligned under shoulders and body straight from head to heels. Hold for 2 counts, then walk hands back and rise up to starting position. Do 10 reps.

JUMP SQUAT TO LUNGE
Works butt and legs

Stand with feet shoulder-width apart, hands in fists at your sides, elbows bent. Squat, then jump up and land in a lunge, right leg in front of left. Jump up and land in a squat, then jump up again and land in a lunge with left leg in front of right. Jump back into the squat again to complete 1 rep. Do 8 reps.

BENTOVER LEG RAISE
Works abs and butt

Hold a dumbbell in each hand at your sides, palms facing legs, and stand with feet hip-width apart.

MY WORKOUT PLAYLIST

Britney Spears

George Michael, "Freedom"

Whitney Houston, "I Wanna Dance with Somebody"

Bruno Mars, "Locked Out of Heaven"

Macklemore, "Thrift Shop"

George Michael, "Father Figure"

Lunge back with your left leg so your right knee is bent 90 degrees and aligned over your ankle. Bend forward from the hips and place weights on the ground in front of your right foot. Stay here and straighten your legs (if you're not flexible enough to do this, place the weights on a low step in front of you.) Keeping your back as straight as possible, raise left leg to hip height behind you, lower toes to the ground, and repeat. Do 10 reps, then switch sides to complete set.

SINGLE-LEG DIP
Works triceps and back

Sit on the edge of a bench (or beach chair). Place hands on the front, next to your hips and extend legs in front of you, feet flexed. Straighten arms, shift your hips off the bench, and raise your left leg a foot off the ground. Keeping leg raised, bend your elbows and lower your hips toward the ground (stay close to the bench; don't let your hips drift forward). Straighten arms and repeat. Do 12 to 15 reps; switch legs halfway through set.

SQUAT FLY
Works shoulders, upper back, butt, and legs

Stand with feet hip-width apart and hold a dumbbell in your right hand at your side, palm facing your leg. Squat and rest your left arm across your thighs. Holding the squat, raise your right arm out to the side to shoulder height. Lower arm and repeat, maintaining the squat the entire time. Do 10 reps; switch sides to complete set.

SCORPION PUSHUP
Works chest, arms, core, and butt

Get in pushup position. Lift your right leg and bend your knee, bringing it outside right shoulder. Keep leg raised as you bend your elbows, lowering your chest toward the ground. Push up and repeat. Do 16 to 20 reps; switch legs halfway through the set.

V CURL
Works biceps and abs

Sit tall and loop the center of a resistance band around the bottom of your feet. Grasp a handle in each hand next to your legs, palms up, and sit back until your abs engage; extend legs a foot off the ground. Holding V position, curl hands toward your shoulders. Extend arms and repeat. Do 12 reps.

MY WORKOUT PLAYLIST

Brooke Burke

Alicia Keys,
"Unthinkable"

Jay-Z featuring Alicia Keys,
"Empire State of Mind"

Black Eyed Peas,
"I Gotta Feeling"

Usher,
"DJ Got Us Fallin' in Love"

Taio Cruz,
"Dynamite"

The Hard-Hitting Workout

When you're on the road (or even when you're at home, for that matter), you usually don't have a lot of time to carve out for monster workout sessions. That's why it's always good to have a plan in your mental back pocket. This workout will get your heart pumping and your muscles scorching—to give you a great fat-burning and body-toning session. Designed by Jillian Michaels, the exercises that follow target multiple muscles so you can maximize your time. As a bonus, there are lots of plyometric moves (powerful jumping exercises) included, which amps up the calorie burn to double-digits-a-minute territory. Do each move for 1 minute in order, then rest for up to 60 seconds. Repeat the entire circuit twice more. (You'll need a pair of 5- to 8-pound dumbbells.)

Gummy
fruit
snacks
260 calories per
2.25-oz bag
YOU ATE IT?
NEGATE IT!
25 minutes
of stair-
climbing

CHAIR POSE JUMP
Works shoulders, back, butt, and legs

Stand with feet together, arms extended at your sides, palms facing thighs. Squat as you raise your arms overhead, then bring them down to your sides (and slightly behind you) as you jump up. Land in starting position and repeat. (If this is too tough, skip the jump and simply squat, rise up, and repeat.)

FALLING PUSHUP
Works shoulders, chest, arms, and core

Get in pushup position with your knees on the ground, shoulders aligned over wrists. Bend elbows out to the sides, forcefully push off the ground, then immediately return to starting position; repeat.

CHEER JUMP
Works core, butt, and legs

Stand with feet together, arms extended at your sides and palms facing your thighs. Jump up, clapping your hands overhead as you separate your legs into an inverted V shape. Land in starting position and repeat.

DEADLIFT TO HAMMER CURL
Works biceps, back, butt, and legs

Stand with feet close together and hold a dumbbell in each hand, arms extended at your sides and palms facing thighs. Keeping your back straight and weights close to your body, bend forward from the hips. Rise up, then bend elbows, curling weights toward your shoulders. Extend arms to starting position and repeat.

JUMPING PLIÉ ROW
Works back, butt, and legs

Stand with feet wide, toes turned out. Hold a dumbbell in each hand, arms extended in front of you and palms facing your body. Bend your knees, then jump as you bend your elbows out to the sides, drawing weights toward your chest until upper arms are parallel to the ground. Land in starting position and repeat.

SUPERMAN ANGEL FLY
Works core

Lie facedown with legs extended hip-width apart on the ground behind you. Hold a dumbbell overhead with both hands, arms extended and palms facing each other; lift arms, legs, and chest. Transfer the weight to your right hand and bring your arms behind your back. Then pass the weight to the left hand and bring arms overhead again, bringing dumbbell to right hand. Continue, lowering chest and legs between each rep if necessary.

ROTATING GOBLET SQUAT
Works butt and legs

Stand with feet shoulder-width apart, toes turned slightly out, and hold a dumbbell with both hands in front of your chest, elbows pointing down. Squat deeply, then jump as you rotate to the left, and land facing the opposite direction. Squat and repeat in opposite direction. Continue, alternating directions.

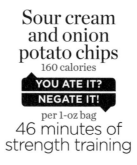

Sour cream
and onion
potato chips
160 calories

YOU ATE IT?
NEGATE IT!

per 1-oz bag
46 minutes of
strength training

HOW TO STAY FIT ON VACATION

Vacations should be the time to splurge a little, but most of us would rather come home with memories, not a few extra pounds. Follow these tips to stay healthy while you're out and about.

✳
Schedule a group class or two at the hotel or a nearby gym. Putting it on your calendar will mean you're more likely to fit it in.

✳
On travel days, pack a bag of nuts, fruits, and string cheese. That will help you avoid airport and rest-stop temptations of the less healthy variety.

✳
Drink lots of water, especially during long flights, to help avoid the grogginess associated with traveling.

The CrossFit Workout

CrossFit has become all the rage—for its combination of strength, endurance, speed, and balance training. The official workouts can look intimidating if you've never tried them. Want to get a taste of what CrossFitters do? Try this workout created by Lauren Plumey. You'll need a pair of 10- to 15-pound dumbbells, as well as a bench, step, or box. Do 16 reps of each move as quickly as possible and do the bear crawl between each exercise.

SINGLE-ARM SNATCH
Works legs, butt, back, shoulders, and arms

Stand with feet wider than shoulders and toes turned out slightly, and place a dumbbell on the floor between your feet. Squat, and grab the dumbbell with your right hand, palm facing behind you. Quickly straighten your legs and rise onto the balls of your feet as you bend your right elbow out to the side, drawing weight toward your shoulder. Bend knees as you flip the weight so your palm faces away from you, and extend your right arm straight overhead. Stand up, then squat, and lower dumbbell toward the ground to return to starting position. Switch arms halfway through set.

BEAR CRAWL
Works entire body

Get on all fours on the ground, then lift your knees. Keeping knees bent, move left foot and hand forward, then step forward with the right foot and hand to complete 1 step. Take 30 steps.

DUMBBELL SWING
Works arms, core, back, butt, and legs

Stand with feet wider than shoulders and toes turned out slightly, and hold the center of a dumbbell with both hands in front of your hips. Squat as you bring the weight between your legs. Quickly rise up as you swing your arms overhead. Return to starting position.

OVERHEAD LUNGE
Works arms, core, butt, and legs

Hold a dumbbell in your left hand and extend your arm overhead, palm facing right. Lunge forward with your right leg, knees bent 90 degrees. Keeping left arm raised, step back to starting position. Lunge forward with your left leg on the next rep. Continue, alternating legs; switch arms halfway through set.

SUMO HIGH PULL
Works shoulders, biceps, back, butt, and legs

Stand with feet wide, toes turned out, and hold a dumbbell in each hand in front of your hips, palms facing behind you. Squat and lower weights between your legs. Rise up as you draw the weights toward your shoulders, elbows high. Return to starting position.

BOX JUMP
Works butt and legs

Stand facing a box, step, or bench (choose a height and width that you can safely clear). Squat and then jump over the object to complete 1 rep. Turn around and repeat in opposite direction.

L STAND
Works arms, chest, core, and back

Kneel on the ground 2 or 3 feet in front of a wall and place hands on the ground in front of you, slightly wider than shoulders. Place your feet on the wall, straighten your legs, and walk your feet up so your body forms an L shape, torso perpendicular to legs. Hold for 15 seconds. (To make it harder, do pushups in this position.)

The Fast Core Workout

To improve your posture, strengthen all of your core muscles, and even help reduce back pain, try this quick plan. Do each move in order; repeat the circuit three times.

SWIMMER

Lie facedown with arms extended overhead, palms on the floor, and legs extended behind you. Raise your left arm and right leg. Return to starting position, then raise right arm and left leg. Continue for 30 seconds, alternating sides.

KNEELING SWIMMER

Get on all fours. Raise your left arm to shoulder height in front of you as you extend your right leg to hip height behind you. Return to starting position. Repeat with opposite arm and leg. Continue for 30 seconds, alternating sides.

PLANK SWIMMER

Get in plank position with hands and toes on the ground. Raise your left arm to shoulder height in front of you as you raise your right leg to hip height behind you. Return to starting position. Repeat with opposite arm and leg. Continue for 30 seconds, alternating sides.

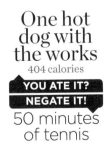

One hot
dog with
the works
404 calories
YOU ATE IT?
NEGATE IT!
50 minutes
of tennis

The Hotel-Treadmill Tone-Up

Don't limit treadmill sessions to only one direction. Walk backward and your hamstrings and glutes will work harder than they do when you move forward; walk sideways and you'll target your inner and outer thighs. Try this multi-directional plan to sneak in a 30-minute session:

0–2 minutes: Walk at an easy pace (incline 1.0)

2–4: Walk briskly

4–6: Side shuffle: Turn left, bend knees slightly, and quickly step to the right with right foot, then bring left foot toward it. Continue for 1 minute, then repeat in opposite direction.

6–8: Walk backward, grasping rails for balance if needed

8–9: Jog

9–10: Lunges: Pause the treadmill, step off, and perform lunges, alternating legs

10–26: Increase the incline by 2.0 and repeat minutes 2–10 twice

26–30: Walk at easy pace

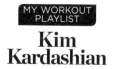

MY WORKOUT PLAYLIST

Kim Kardashian

Black Eyed Peas,
"I Gotta Feeling"

Lady GaGa,
"Telephone"

Beyoncé,
"If I Were a Boy"

Anything by
J.Lo!

Get in the Swim of Things

Too hot to train outside? Or maybe you're looking to mix things up? Swimming is one of the best exercises you can do, as it works every muscle in your body and fries the fries right off you (not that you're having many of them, except maybe in your cheat meal!). In fact, it burns up to 230 calories every 20 minutes. But for those who haven't done much swimming since their kiddie summers, it can be a daunting task. Here are some basics to get you going in the water:

Workouts: You can do steady-state swims and reap tons of benefits, but mixing up your routine can help add variety, and including intervals will increase your calorie burn. One example of how you can do it:

200m (meters) warmup

4 x 50m at fast pace (rest for about 20 seconds after each 50m)

2 x 50m with kickboard (same rest as above)

2 x 50m with upper-body strokes only, no kicking (same rest as above)

400m at slightly faster pace than warmup, but one you can maintain for this distance

200m cooldown

Basics of Breathing: When your face is submerged, slowly and steadily exhale through your nose or mouth (holding your breath increases pressure in your lungs, which can make your muscles tense and cause legs to sink, which slows you down). Try to practice breathing to both sides, taking a breath every three strokes.

Check Your Form: Look into a pool where a bunch of people are doing laps and you'll see as many different swimming forms as you do bathing suits. But if you can use proper form, you'll go faster and swim more efficiently. Bottom line: If you can get your butt and legs up, you'll swim through the water, rather than dragging your lower body against it. Some ways to perfect form:

Palms: As you draw your arm back, cup your hand like a paddle to pull the water, to help propel you.

Elbow: As your arm comes out of the water, bend your elbow so it points to the sky.

Head: Keep your eyes looking down at the bottom of the pool, not out in front of you. Dropping your head helps lift your hips.

Legs: Slightly bend your knees. Focus on using your entire leg (originating the motion from your hips) for the kick.

Body: Rotate your whole body slightly toward your extended arm.

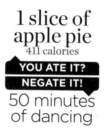

1 slice of
apple pie
411 calories

YOU ATE IT?
NEGATE IT!

50 minutes
of dancing

NO ROOM FOR LAPS?

If your hotel pool is smaller than a kitchen, it may not give you enough space to get in a swim, but you can get a great workout by running in deep water. Researchers in India found that deep-water running improved endurance on land. It burns mega calories, improves your endurance, and (thanks to the resistance provided by water) sculpts your legs, butt, and core. You can strap on a flotation belt or hold onto a foam noodle (put it behind your back or hold it out in front of you). In the water, start jogging, bringing your knees no higher than your hips and kicking your rear foot toward your butt.

The Jump-Rope Workout

If you buy only one piece of equipment, make it a jump rope. This portable gear may be light, but it's a cardio heavy-hitter. Jumping rope burns about 10 calories a minute, while strengthening your heart. Plus it tones your legs to boot.

0–2 minutes: Lunge, alternating legs

2–5: Jump rope, easy pace

5–6: Squat

6–8: Jump rope, moderate pace

8–9: Mountain climbers

9–10: Jump rope, fast

10–20: Repeat minutes 0–10

20–22: Lunge, alternating legs

22–25: Jump rope, easy pace

MY WORKOUT PLAYLIST

Audrina Patridge

Edward Maya,
"Stereo Love"

Iration,
"Time Bomb"

Black Eyed Peas,
"Just Can't Get Enough"

Lykke Li,
"Get Some"

The John Butler Trio,
"What You Want"

The Walking Workout

Sometimes, you just may not have the time or energy to get through a high-intensity workout. When you feel this way, try the simplest form of cardio there is: walking. The activity can be done anywhere (perfect for when you're visiting a new city). Want to take your stroll up a notch? Try this plan. It gets your heart pumping and includes intensity-boosting shuffles that help target your outer thighs.

0–5 minutes: Walk at easy to moderate pace

5–8: Walk fast

8–9: Side-step shuffle

9–10: Walk at a moderate pace

10–25: Repeat minutes 5–10 three times

25–26: Walk as fast as you can

26–28: Walk at a moderate pace

28–34: Repeat minutes 25–28 twice

34–36: Walk fast

36–40: Cool down at a moderate pace

MY WORKOUT PLAYLIST

Rosario Dawson

Gil-Scott Heron, "Must Be Something"

Van Morrison, "The Way Young Lovers Do"

Marvin Gaye, "I Want You"

Joni Mitchell, "All I Want"

Tom Waits, "Step Right Up"

The TRX Workout

One of our favorite pieces of exercise equipment is the TRX Suspension Trainer. Functioning a little bit like gymnastics rings, the trainer allows you to use your body weight and gravity to work your muscles in all kinds of positions. You can hit every inch with this one piece of equipment— which makes it perfect for home or travel. You can buy one for about $200, but many gyms now have them set up. Ready to try the TRX? Do each exercise for 30 seconds in order, moving at a slow, controlled pace. Repeat the series twice.

PUSHUP
Works chest, arms, and core

Stand facing away from the TRX with feet shoulder-width apart. Hold handles at chest height in front of you, arms extended and palms facing the floor. With your body aligned from head to heels, shift weight to the balls of your feet and bend your elbows. Push up to return to the starting position.

INVERTED ROW
Works back, biceps, and core

Lie faceup under the TRX with knees bent and feet on the floor. Hold the handles over your chest, arms extended and palms facing each other. Bend elbows, pulling your torso up toward your hands. Extend arms to starting position.

TRICEPS EXTENSION
Works triceps and core

Stand facing away from the TRX with feet hip-width apart. Lean forward and grasp handles in front of your face, elbows bent

90 degrees and palms facing away from you. Extend your arms, then bend your elbows to return to the starting position.

HIGH CURL
Works biceps and core

Stand facing the TRX with feet hip-width apart. Hold handles at chest height in front of you, arms extended and palms facing up, and lean back. Bend your elbows, curling hands toward your head. Return to starting position.

LUNGE
Works core, butt, and legs

Stand facing away from the TRX with left foot on both foot cradles and hands on your hips. (Both legs should be extended.) Bend knees until your right thigh is parallel to the floor; rise up to starting position and repeat. Switch legs to complete set.

KNEE DRIVE
Works core, butt, and legs

Stand facing the TRX and hold handles high in front of you, palms facing each other. Bend your left knee 90 degrees, shifting weight to your right leg. Bend your right knee. Then rise up onto the ball of your right foot as you lift your left knee to hip height in front of you and bend elbows, pulling handles toward your chest. Return to starting position and repeat. Switch sides to complete set.

HAMSTRING PULL-IN
Works core and butt

Lie faceup with your heels in the TRX's foot cradles, legs extended and arms straight out to the sides in a T position, palms on floor. Lift hips so body is aligned from shoulders to heels. Bend knees, pulling handles toward you. Extend legs to starting position.

The Romantic Getaway Workout

Say you and your partner have planned a nice getaway—sightseeing, dinners, a show. All wonderful, but there's also nothing wrong with squeezing in a little time to get sweaty together. Besides being good for your body, it's also good for your mood and your relationship. Try this fun workout that's built for two. Do each move for 1 minute, then repeat the entire circuit once or twice more.

MIRROR SQUAT
Works butt and legs

Stand facing each other, about a foot apart, with feet slightly wider than shoulders. Clasp each other's hands at chest height in front of you and squat until your thighs are parallel to the floor, then rise up to starting position.

PARTNER PRESS
Works shoulders, chest, triceps, and core

Have your partner lie faceup with legs bent and feet on the floor. Get in plank position above him, with your hands on the floor beside your partner's shoulders; have him place his hands on your shoulders, elbows bent. Bend your elbows, and push up as your partner extends his arms, lifting you. Return to starting position and repeat for 30 seconds, then switch positions for the next 30.

SIDE SHUFFLE
Works butt and legs

Stand facing each other with about a foot between you, feet hip-width apart. Bend elbows, raise arms to shoulder height in front of you, and press your palms against your partner's. Bend knees and step to the right as your partner steps to the left, then step back. Continue shuffling to the right for 30 seconds, then repeat in opposite direction.

POWER PUNCH
Works shoulders, chest, and back

Stand facing each other with feet staggered, left in front of right, and knees slightly bent. Hold your right hand at chest height in front of you, elbow bent; your partner extends his right arm. Clasp your right hand and place your left hand on your hips. Extend your right arm forward as your partner resists. Bend elbow and repeat for 15 seconds, then switch (partner punches and you resist) for 15 seconds. Repeat on opposite side.

TOWEL TWIST
Works core, butt, and legs

Hold a towel in front of your belly and stand facing away from your partner, feet shoulder-width apart and knees bent. Twist to the left as your partner twists to the right, and hand him the towel. Rotate to opposite side and grab the towel from your partner. Continue alternating sides and handing the towel to each other.

PLEASURE TO MEET YOU
Works shoulders, chest, and core

Get in pushup position (either on toes or knees), head-to-head and about arm's length apart. Bend your elbows, lowering your chest toward the floor. Push up, lift right arm, and shake each other's hand. Return to starting position and repeat, this time shaking left hands. Continue, alternating hands on each rep.

PULL TOGETHER
Works back, abs, butt, and legs

Lie faceup with knees bent and feet on the floor; your partner stands over your hips and squats. Extend your arms and grasp his left hand with your right, and his right with your left. Bend your elbows, pulling yourself toward your partner. Lower to starting position. Continue for 30 seconds, then switch positions, and repeat.

RESCUE ME
Works shoulders, arms, back, and core

Sit facing each other with knees bent and feet touching, each holding one end of a towel. Your partner lies faceup on the floor (the towel should be taut) and places his right hand above his left, then left above right, pulling himself up until he's sitting. Return to starting position and repeat for 30 seconds. Then switch positions (you lie down) and repeat.

HIGH FIVE
Works entire body

Lie faceup with knees bent and feet on the floor, toe-to-toe with your partner. Sit up as you place your left hand on the floor beside your left hip and extended your right arm in front of you, touching his right palm. Stand up, pushing against each other, jump, then high-five each other. Return to starting position and repeat with opposite hand.

DRUM LINE
Works shoulders, back, arms, butt, and legs

Stand facing each other, about 2 feet apart, with feet wider than shoulders and knees bent. Your partner holds a towel taut at belly height horizontally in front of him. Bend elbows and bring your hands in front of your face, palms facing each other. "Chop" the towel with your left hand across the length for 15 seconds, then repeat with right hand for 15 seconds. Switch positions with your partner and repeat.

The Playground Workout

Stuck in a spot with no gym, or just want a change of pace? Walk on over to the nearest park and use the playground equipment to get a total-body burn. You can do this plan on its own as a strength workout or midway through a walk or run. Do 12 to 15 reps of each move back to back. Repeat the circuit two or three times.

PRONE PULLUP
Works back, biceps, and core

Grasp a bar or rope (the lower it is, the more challenging the move is) with hands shoulder-width apart, palms facing away from you. Walk feet forward until arms and legs are extended and chest is under hands; tighten your abs so your body is straight from your head to heels. Keeping abs tight and head in line with your spine, bend your elbows, pulling your chest toward the bar. Straighten arms and repeat.

HANGING KNEE LIFT
Works arms and abs

Grab a rope or bar that's about 5- to 7-feet high with hands shoulder-width apart and palms facing away from you. Hang from it with your arms straight (if your feet are still on the ground, bend your knees). Pull knees toward your chest, then slowly extend legs, and repeat.

DECLINE PUSHUP TO SIDE PLANK
Works shoulders, chest, triceps, and core

Get in plank position with feet on the end of a slide, wrists under shoulders, abs tight, and head in line with spine. Bend your elbows, lowering your chest the toward the ground; straighten arms and

Take Your Cardio Outside

Summer is a great time to mix up your workouts. These fun outdoor activities, complete with some tips to help you master them, can help you burn extra calories while sculpting your muscles at the same time.

Kayaking
(burns up to 600 calories an hour)

❋ Always wear a flotation device.

❋ To get in, place the kayak halfway in the water, straddle the seat, then push off from shore. On a dock, squat before sitting—lowering your center of gravity helps prevent falling.

❋ Sit up straight. Reclining strains your back, while leaning forward can cause your neck and shoulders to tense.

❋ As you paddle, bend your elbows 90 degrees and rotate your entire torso. Great core workout!

❋ To steer right, sweep the paddle away from your kayak on the left side.

Hiking
(burns up to 500 calories an hour)

❋ Make sure you have enough water, sunscreen, a snack, a phone, a waterproof jacket, and a small flashlight (just in case!).

❋ Buddy up when you can. If you're going solo, make sure you tell someone your route and when you plan to get back.

❋ Lean forward slightly when walking uphill, but stay loose and flexible when hiking downhill. Consider using trekking poles, which can reduce impact on your joints.

Cycling
(burns up to 700 calories an hour)

❋ Wear a helmet and have a bike mechanic adjust your handlebars and saddle for a proper fit.

❋ As soon as your pace decreases, switch to a lower gear until you're working at moderate intensity again. When you find yourself pedaling too fast, shift up to a higher gear.

❋ Start riding in a park or neighborhood before taking it out on the road. Follow all traffic laws as if you were driving a car.

Trail Running
(burns up to 600 calories)

❋ Assume it will take longer to cover the same distance than you would on the treadmill or road.

❋ Take small steps to help you stay steady on uneven ground. Walk whenever it gets too rocky or rooty.

❋ Focus your eyes a few feet in front of you to avoid objects, and lift your feet up a little higher than usual to have them clear any unforeseen obstacles.

repeat. Do all reps, then rotate your body to the left and extend left arm straight up in line with your shoulders. Hold for 5 counts, then return to the starting position and repeat rotation and arm raise on the opposite side.

BENCH DIP
Works triceps and core

Sit on a bench with knees bent. Place hands on the front edge with your fingers facing forward, slide hips off bench, and straighten your arms (don't lock elbows). Extend left leg in front of you, thighs even. Bend elbows behind you, lowering your hips toward the ground and keeping them close to the bench. Press up and repeat. Switch sides (raise right leg) halfway through the set. For more of a challenge, extend your balancing leg in front of you.

STEP HOP
Works butt and legs

Stand with your right foot on a step and left foot on the step below it or on the ground. Bend elbows at your sides and squat. Push off your right foot as you jump up, lifting your left leg out to the left side. Land in starting position and repeat. Switch sides to complete set. If you don't want to jump, simply lift your left leg up to the side as you rise out of the squat.

FLYING SIDE LUNGE
Works shoulders, butt, and legs

Hold a ring or rope in each hand overhead and stand with feet hip-width apart. Keeping shoulders down (no hunching) and feet parallel, lunge to the left with your left leg. Continue holding the rings as you bend your left knee deeper. Push off your left foot to step back to starting position (focus on using your legs more than your arms) and repeat. Switch sides to complete the set.

The Ball and Band Workout

With nothing more than a stability ball and a resistance band or tube, you can sculpt your body in all the right places. The ball challenges your balance, making your core work especially hard to stabilize you. And the tension in bands stays constant as you bend and extend, keeping your muscles fully engaged the entire time. Try this workout, designed by SPRI master trainer Abbie Appel. Do each move in order for 1 minute, without resting in between.

SLIDE-OUT SQUAT
Works butt and legs

Stand with your right shin on a stability ball and left foot on the ground beside it, hands on your hips. Squat as you push your right leg out to the side, rolling the ball to the right. Rise up to starting position and repeat. Switch sides after 30 seconds.

DOUBLE RAISE
Works shoulders and outer thighs

Stand with your left foot on the center of a resistance tube and hold a handle in each hand in front of your thighs, palms facing each other. Raise your left arm to shoulder height to the side as you lift your right leg out to the side. Lower arms and leg to starting position and repeat. Switch sides after 30 seconds.

BALANCE CURL
Works biceps and core

Stand with left foot on the center of a resistance tube and hold a handle at your sides, palms facing away from you. Raise your right leg behind you. Bend elbows, curling your hands toward your shoulders. Keeping right leg raised, extend your arms to starting position and repeat. Switch legs after 30 seconds.

BALL CIRCLE
Works shoulders and core

Get in plank position with your forearms on a stability ball, fingers clasped. Keeping the rest of your body still, use your elbows to move the ball in a circle to the right. Switch direction (move in a circle to the left) after 30 seconds.

Summer Sports Spectacular

Go ahead and jump into your favorite summer activities. Beach volleyball, for example, can burn up to 550 calories an hour. Plus, the stop-start action engages your core and lower body. Or try surfing or stand-up paddleboarding. Because balancing on water is so challenging, these activities sculpt all the stabilizing muscles in your core while blasting up to six calories a minute. (The benefits, by the way, aren't just physical. Research shows that you get a bigger mood boost from exercising in the water than in other environments.)

To stand up on a paddleboard:

✳ Choose a board that's 10 to 12 feet long and 30 inches wide. It should be light and narrow, but still stable.

✳ Keep your eyes up as you try to stand. Looking down throws off your center of balance and can lead you to take an unplanned dip. Your body will follow where your eyes go.

✳ Stand in the middle of the board, feet hip-width apart and knees bent. The rougher the water, the deeper you should squat.

✳ As you paddle, engage your core and rotate your torso. That will help with propulsion and balance.

HINGE EXTENSION
Works triceps and core

Stand with your left foot on the center of a resistance tube and hold a handle in each hand at your sides, elbows bent 90 degrees and palms facing up. Shift weight to left foot, extending your right leg on the ground behind you and your arms straight back. Return to starting position and repeat. Switch legs after 30 seconds.

BOOTY KICK
Works butt

Get on all fours with the center of a resistance tube wrapped twice around your left foot and a handle anchored by each hand; raise your left foot off the ground. Extend your left leg to hip height behind you. Bend your left knee to return to starting position and repeat. Switch legs after 30 seconds.

ROTATING FLY
Works shoulders, abs, and back

Sit with knees slightly bent and the center of a resistance tube wrapped around your feet. Hold a handle in each hand, your left arm bent at 90 degrees at your sides with palm facing up and right arm extended in front of your shoulder, elbow slightly bent and palm facing left. Pull your right arm out to the side. Keeping arms and legs still, rotate shoulders to the right. Twist back to center, then return right arm to starting position and repeat. Switch sides after 30 seconds.

MY WORKOUT PLAYLIST

Vanessa Hudgens

Black Eyed Peas,
"The Time"

Deadmau5,
"Ghost N Stuff"

Bassnectar,
"Bass Head"

T.A.T.U.,
"Not Gonna Get Us"

Yeah Yeah Yeahs,
"Heads Will Roll"

The Fighting Words Workout

This workout is from Annika Kahn, creator of Jungshin Fitness, which combines kickboxing and yoga principles. Do 3 sets of each move in order. You'll need a 1- or 3-pound wooden practice sword.

POWER STRIKE
Works shoulders, arms, back, butt, and legs

Hold the sword in front of your hips, pointing down, with your right hand on the sword's ridge and left hand just above it. Lunge forward with your right foot and turn left toes out. Inhale as you raise your arms overhead, bending your elbows so the sword is parallel to your back. Exhale as you rotate your torso to the left and extend arms, striking sword down to the left. Raise the sword to starting position and repeat, rotating to the right, to complete 1 rep. Do 10 reps; switch legs halfway through the set.

FIGHTER STANCE
Works core, butt, and legs

Hold sword with right hand on the ridge in front of your chest, left hand open and above left shoulder. Stand with feet wide, knees slightly bent, and inhale. Exhale as you step your right foot back at a diagonal to the left and squat. Step back to the starting position; repeat. Do 10 reps, then switch legs to complete set.

ROUNDHOUSE KICK
Works core, butt, and legs

Hold sword with right hand on the ridge in front of your chest, left hand open and above left shoulder, and stand with feet together.

Inhale as you raise your right knee to hip height out to the side, foot flexed, and lean torso to the left, then exhale as you extend your right leg. Return to the starting position and immediately repeat. Do 10 reps; switch legs to complete set.

JUNGSHIN ABS
Works shoulders, arms, and core

Sit with knees bent, ankles crossed, and feet on the ground. Hold sword at chest height in front of you, pointing down. Inhale as you bring your arms overhead, bending elbows so sword is parallel to your spine. Exhale as you lean back and uncross your ankles, extending arms and legs at a 45-degree angle in front of you. Return to starting position and repeat for 30 seconds.

KNEELING MEDITATION
Works shoulders, arms, and back

Hold sword in front of you, pointing down, and kneel with the tops of your feet on the ground. Inhale as you raise your arms overhead, bending your elbows so the sword is behind your back. Exhale as you return to starting position.

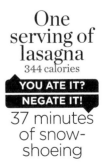

One
serving of
lasagna
344 calories
YOU ATE IT?
NEGATE IT!
37 minutes
of snow-
shoeing

The 10-Minute Fat Blaster

You don't need any equipment for this one, which means it's perfect for when you're on the road or you want to get in a quick sweat session while the relatives are prepping the grill. Perform each move at a fast pace for 1 minute without resting in between. Repeat.

CROSS JACK
Works shoulders and legs

Stand with feet wide and arms extended at shoulder height out to sides, palms facing the ground. Jump and cross your right arm

---

SUPERHERO MOVES

Fancy yourself as a little more advanced? Ready for a new challenge? Amp up the intensity with these variations on three familiar moves.

Instead of a regular pushup...

Instead of a regular squat...

Instead of a plank...

DONKEY KICK PUSHUP
Works chest, triceps, core, and legs

Get in plank position with wrists aligned under shoulders. Bend elbows straight back behind you, lowering your chest toward the ground. Push up, then jump feet toward your hands and kick them up into the air, bringing your heels toward your butt. Jump feet back to starting position and repeat.

HARDCORE SQUAT
Works core, butt, and legs

Stand with feet shoulder-width apart, hands behind your ears, and squat. Rise up as you raise your right knee to hip height in front of you and rotate your shoulders to the right. Twist back to center as you jump up and kick your left foot forward. Return to starting position; repeat on opposite side to complete 1 rep.

BREAK-DANCER
Works arms, core, and legs

Get on all fours, knees and heels lifted. Hop feet to the right, extending your left leg to the right as you reach for the left foot with your right hand. Immediately repeat in opposite direction. Continue, alternating sides.

over left at shoulder height in front of you as you cross your right foot over left. Jump back to starting position and repeat, crossing opposite arm and foot. Continue, alternating sides.

PLANK HEEL TOUCH
Works shoulders, chest, triceps, abs, and lower back

Get in plank position with feet shoulder-width apart. Bring your right heel toward your butt as you reach back and touch it with your left hand. Return to starting position and repeat with opposite arm and leg. Continue, alternating sides.

SKATER SQUAT
Works butt and legs

Stand with feet together and arms at your sides, hands in fists. Jump to the left as you extend your left arm behind you and right fist toward your chin, landing on your left foot with your right leg raised behind you. Immediately squat, then repeat in opposite direction. Continue, alternating sides.

DROP-SQUAT PUNCH
Works shoulders, arms, back, butt, and legs

Stand with feet together, elbows bent, and hands in fists under chin. Jump feet out wide and squat as you punch forward with your right hand. Jump back to starting position and repeat, punching with the left hand. Continue, alternating sides.

JUMP LUNGE
Works butt and legs

Lunge forward with left leg, elbows bent and hands in fists, right hand in front of your chest and left hand at your hip. Jump as you switch legs and arms, landing in a lunge with right foot in front. Continue, switching legs every jump.

The Pilates-Inspired Workout

This Synergy 7 System workout, designed by Pilates instructor Kit Rich and master energy trainer Joshua Farahnik, combines the benefits of strength training with meditation sessions. Do each move for 1 minute in order, breathing through your nose and out through your mouth.

FLYING SUMO
Works butt and legs

Stand with feet wide, toes turned out slightly. Inhale as you squat until your thighs are parallel to the floor, and extend arms overhead, fingers spread wide. Exhale as you rise up and jump. Return to starting position.

THIRD-EYE CLIMB
Works chest, arms, and core

Get in plank position, hands slightly wider than your shoulders. Lift your right leg to hip height behind you and inhale. Exhale as you round your spine, push your hips up, and pull your right knee toward your forehead. Hold for 1 second, then return to starting position and repeat with opposite leg. Continue, alternating sides.

BOWING CRANE
Works back

Lie facedown with elbows bent and palms pressed together on top of your head; inhale. Exhale as you lift your shoulders and chest. Inhale as you lower to starting position. Exhale as you open your arms out to your sides, palms facing forward. Inhale as you return to the starting position.

CREATIVE CRUNCH
Works abs

Lie faceup with knees bent and slightly wider than shoulders, feet together on the floor. Place hands behind your head and tilt your chin so you're looking at the ceiling; inhale. Exhale as you crunch up, squeezing your knees together. Return to the starting position.

AB GOODNESS
Works abs

Lie faceup with arms and legs extended on the floor, heels together, and toes turned out, palms facing ceiling; inhale. Exhale as you lift your head, shoulders, and arms, and raise legs at a diagonal in front of you. Pump arms up and down 7 times, exhaling with each pump. Lower to starting position.

WATERING ELEPHANT
Works entire body

Get in a side plank position on your right elbow. Inhale as you reach under the right side of your body with your left arm. Exhale as you rotate your left shoulder back, reaching your left arm behind you. Return to starting position. Switch sides after 30 seconds.

TABLE SWING
Works arms, core, butt, and legs

Sit with hands aligned under your shoulders, knees bent, and feet on the floor in front of you. Push hips forward and up, getting into tabletop position; inhale. Exhale as you straighten your legs and push your hips back between your hands, keeping your butt off the floor if you can. Inhale as you return to tabletop position.

CHAPTER 11

Finding Your Best Bathing Suit

How to Make the Most of Your New Body

So let's say you've been following our plan, eating your BEACH foods, sweating it out, and changing right before your very eyes. Now it's time to change again—right into your bikini!

Maybe once you dreaded trying on bathing suits—because of all the angst and stress you felt trying to hide what you didn't like. But now, you're going to embrace it. You have confidence. You have a body that you love. You have all the eating and exercise strategies that have given you energy *and* attitude.

Now all you need? Your bikini.

When you go shopping, it's all about matching a style and shape with your style and shape.

Remember, a bikini body isn't about having one ideal figure. It's about having *your* best bikini body. And it's not about one particular swimsuit that you need to fit into, it's about finding the look that makes you happy, comfortable, and confident. Though it's up to you whether you like quiet or loud, solid or stripes, skimpy or conservative, I have been helping women look great in bikinis for years, and I can pass on some essential tips for finding the one that will play up the positives and give you confidence in areas you're less crazy about. Use your body type as a guide to pick your most flattering swimwear.

YOUR BODY TYPE

Athletic: Your best bet is to look for swimsuits that create the illusion of curves. Opt for pretty prints and girly details like fringe and ruffles to help soften your silhouette and add some inches to your shape.

A DAY OR TWO BEFORE YOU SHOP FOR A SUIT, APPLY SELF-TANNER.

It will help reduce the green cast of the fluorescent lighting that's commonly used in fitting rooms, which can make even Selena Gomez look like Gomez Addams. That means you'll get a truer sense of how the bikini will look on you outdoors.

Busty: If you're large-chested, look for halter styles, which lend ample support. Wide straps and built-in underwires are two uplifters that won't leave you hanging. Also look for graphic-print bottoms with high-cut legs that can bring attention to a lean lower half. And structured, bra-like cups help defy gravity.

Apple: If you have a little extra weight around your tummy, use draping and certain cuts to visually take inches off your waistline. Look for suits with side ruching, which helps create the appearance of a narrow waist; and built in high tech stretch and control paneling lend support to help tuck you in.

Pear: If you're larger below than on top, one-pieces with deep-V necklines divert attention from fuller hips and help lengthen your torso. If you go for a bikini, a subtly ruffled or skirted bottom helps hide saddlebags. You can also try an asymmetrical top to help downplay fuller hips, or a cleavage-enhancing overlay to draw eyes away from your lower body.

Curvy: Look for suits with all-over ruching to play up an hourglass shape and give you a beautiful retro-vibe. If wearing a two-piece, full coverage cups are a must and bottoms with fold-over waistbands won't pinch and create the dreaded muffin top. You can also try a tankini with a blousy fit, which will skim over (and not squeeze) a pooch.

A great tip: Assess your swimsuit at home. Due to that unflattering and artificial department store lighting, it's smart buy and then try on at home. You'll get a more accurate read of how you look and feel in the suit. So simply buy, try, then return the options that don't work.

Extend Your Bikini's Lifespan

Rinse after every wearing. Run cold water over your swimsuit as soon as you take it off to help remove the salt and chlorine, which can damage the fabric.

Remove excess water by gently squeezing. Wringing or twisting can cause your suit to lose its shape.

Handwash it in cool water. Chemical detergents and the agitation of a washer can break down fabric. If you use a machine, use an all-natural detergent on a gentle cycle.

Lay it flat to dry. The high heat from a dryer destroys the elastic fibers—air-dry to help keep its shape.

Here are a few more summer tips I affectionately call "shore things":

Feel-Good Flips

We want your feet to look and feel great in your summer get-ups, but flip-flops and sandals can lead to some foot problems (see page 249 for foot-care guidance). Here are some tips for making sure you find a pair that's both stylish and supportive.

Support: Look for a visible arch formation. It's also best if there's a little padded cradle for your heel. The toe end should slope upward a bit to help you grip while walking.

Flexibility: The sandals should have a slight bend to them, so they can help with the walking gait (by helping your foot push off the ground). But they shouldn't be too floppy. If you can fold them in half with your hands, put them back on the shelf.

Traction: Tread patterns will help keep you grounded, so you're less likely to slip on slick surfaces.

Sexy Shades

When shopping for a new pair of sunglasses, choose ones that cover the entire eye area and block 100 percent of UVA/UVB rays (check the label). The best lenses: Gray or green tints for driving, and bronze or amber if you often spend time by the water. To maximize your look, try to complement the shape of your face with the shape of the shades. A quick guide:

Oval face: With your balanced proportions, you can rock practically any frames, so experiment with the latest trends.

Heart-shaped face: To offset a broader forehead and narrow jawline, choose a classic aviator or semi-rimless style.

Round face: Rectangular or geometric sunglasses help to create the illusion of a slimmer face shape.

Square face: Shades that have gently rounded edges instantly soften and flatter more angular features.

Cool Cover-Ups

Now that you have your bikini body, there's no need for cover-ups, right? Not true. Even the best bikini-bodied women know that there's a time and place for strutting in suits. So how to pick a chic and sexy cover-up to look your best as you stroll through the sand, the deck, the lobby, or down to the ice machine? Opt for a universally flattering style: One that's knee-length and cinches just below the bust—creates shape and forgives all figure flaws. As a bonus, some of them even come with UV-protective properties to further shield skin from the sun's damaging rays, so you'll not only look good right then and there, but also for many years to come.

Note: Be careful with white fabrics. When they get wet, they'll become transparent, leaving you unprotected from sun rays.

Top It Off

Your body isn't the only thing that needs protection from the sun. Your head does, too. Consider a wide-brimmed hat, or shield your scalp with this simple trick:

✳ **Step One:** Wrap a long rectangular scarf around the back of your head, leaving an equal amount of fabric on each side.

✳ **Step Two:** Bring each end to the top of your head, and firmly twist around twice.

✳ **Step Three:** Tightly tie the end in a knot at the nape of your neck to secure it. Voila! Chic and shielded.

Suit Yourself!

The flattering swimwear featured on these pages will have you looking (and feeling) fabulous—no matter your body type. So go on, hit that beach with confidence!

Curvy   If you are curvy, look for...

BODY SHAPERS

✳ A classic retro cut with allover ruching plays up an hourglass shape.

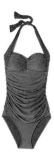

✳Side ties create the illusion of a smaller midsection.

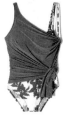

✳ Full-coverage cups hold you in; a foldover waistband won't pinch.

Pear   If you are pear-shaped, look for...

HIP SLIMMERS

✳ A padded bandeau and hipster-cut bottoms help balance your proportions.

✳ In a brightly patterned top, your upper half will be the focal point.

✳ Subtly ruffled or skirted bottoms look cute and help to camouflage saddlebags.

Apple If you are apple-shaped, look for...

TUMMY TRIMMERS

✹ High-rise bottoms have a toning effect, while a high-cut leg elongates.

✹ Suits with hidden control panels will help whittle your middle.

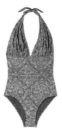

✹ Angled stripes add definition and flatter your midsection.

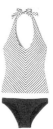

Athletic If your build is athletic, look for...

CURVE CREATORS

✹ Fringe, ruffles, and bows add inches to a straighter shape.

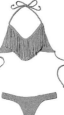

✹ Cutouts and bold color-blocking give the illusion of curves.

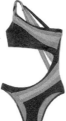

✹ Adjustable straps and padding have a push-up effect.

Busty If you are busty, look for...

UPLIFTERS

✹ Thanks to wide straps and underwire, you won't be left hanging.

✹ Cups in actual sizes ensure an accurate, bra-like fit.

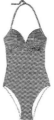

✹ Lighter, patterned bottoms draw the eye downward.

CHAPTER 12

A Bikini Body Grooming Guide

Prepare Your New Body for Showing Off

If you were to envision your Bikini Body Diet lifestyle as a pyramid, we can all agree what would be at the base of it: Nutrition. Without a smart eating plan, frankly, it doesn't matter how much exercise you do or what color suit you're wearing: You're probably not going to look or feel your best.

Next up on the pyramid: Exercise. A strong plan that combines cardio and resistance training helps burn the fat and build muscle. Together, they hold everything else up.

But the pyramid doesn't end there. At the very top, of course, are the fine points—the points that perhaps take a little less time but can go a long way in completing your new look. That's where grooming comes in.

Of course, there are plenty of tricks I can reveal to you to hide this or show off that. But what I'm talking about is using beauty tips to accentuate what you've already developed through smart eating, persistnece, and exercise.

Before I was the editor-in-chief of *Shape,* I was a beauty and fashion director for more than a decade. That experience taught me that no matter how lean and fit you are—and especially, if you aren't—smart beauty tricks and savvy styling can make an enormous difference. They're the finishing touches that will have you feeling more confident and sexier than ever. Trust me: These are the tricks of the trade I've learned from the best celebrity fashion stylists and beauty gurus over the years. Now get ready to wear your suit with pride.

Shape Up Your Bikini Line

A groomed bikini line is a must. (I get Brazilians at NYC's Uni K Salon.) Here, a few key points for going bare:

Shaving is the most traditional way to remove hair. Be sure to use a razor specifically for this sensitive area. Always start with a moisturizing gel to avoid razor burn; and shave upward. Note: You'll need to shave every few days to keep stubble at bay.

For de-fuzzing that lasts up to a month, opt for waxing like I do. Though it hurts a bit during the process, it lasts three to four weeks.

Alternatively, try a depilatory: Simply smooth it onto your bikini line, wait a few minutes and then rinse away. (Always test on a small part of your forearm first to make sure you don't have an allergic reaction.)

Whether you shave, use a depilatory, or wax, ingrown hairs can crop up—triggered by curly hairs growing back into the surrounding skin. Skin will then grow over that hair, and that's what causes the little red bumps. Whatever you do, don't try to pluck them with tweezers, which could lead to an infection or a scar. Instead, spread on an AHA formula, which will clear away cells that clog follicles but also contains an anti-inflammatory that can soothe irritation.

If you're especially prone to ingrown hairs or are looking for a long-lasting de-fuzzing treatment, consider laser hair removal.

And don't forget about your legs! With all of those leg-tightening workouts, you're well on your way to giving your legs the shape you want. But there's another detail that can make even the sexiest of legs even sexier for a silky look and feel. Be sure to wax, shave, or use a depilatory before baring skin, and moisturize daily.

Ditch Dimples

Dreaded cellulite. Those pesky little patches of puckered skin that we ALL battle (I know I do!) can make you want to run for cover on the beach. While sadly there is no "magic cure" for it, these are the tricks you can use to help even things out.

Brush work: Joanna Vargas, an amazing celebrity facialist, taught me that dry-brushing every morning before you shower helps tone and firm skin. Find a natural-bristle brush and use long upward stokes on dry skin. Begin at your feet and work up toward your heart. Give jiggly bits some extra effort. Dry-brushing helps increase blood flow and stimulates lymphatic drainage, which is the number one weapon against puckering. Added bonus: It sloughs away dull skin and leaves you feeling baby soft. You'll see results in just one week.

Kick some butt with caffeine: While the latest anti-cellulite creams won't magically make you look like Gisele, they will provide a tightening effect that will give you an instant lift. Look for those containing caffeine. A jolt of java on bumpy bits helps remove water in the connective tissues and de-bloats the skin so cellulite is less noticeable. To get the biggest caffeine boost, vigorously massage the cream into your thighs, stomach, bottom, and upper arms. The harder you rub, the deeper the ingredients penetrate and the sleeker you'll look. Try this before bed every night.

SURPRISING WAYS TO SAVE YOUR SKIN

✳
**MAINTAIN
A HEALTHY
WEIGHT**
Several studies have suggested a link between obesity and skin cancer, possibly caused by inflammatory reactions to the skin that are associated with higher blood sugar levels.

✳
**EAT
POMEGRANATES**
They're high in antioxidants, which fight against the damaging substances created by UV light.

✳
**USE CURRY
IN YOUR
BEACH FOODS**
The yellow spice contains turmeric, a compound that has been shown to inhibit the development of skin cancer.

✳
**ADD
ANOTHER
SUPPLEMENT**
Research from the University of Colorado shows that milk thistle extract might help damaged skin repair itself.

Embrace Sunless Tanning

My absolute number one confidence booster and beauty splurge that helps me brave my bikini is a spray tan. (More on protecting your skin from the sun on page 254.) Darker objects appear smaller; getting a spray tan or using a sunless tanner at home will help camouflage cellulite and make you look sculpted and slimmer. Believe me, a golden glow is like a magic wand that makes flaws disappear. Not to mention that it's the only safe tan out there.

There are two types of spray tans: Airbrush tans, where an aesthetician personally mists sunless tanner onto your skin, and automatic spray-tanning booths, which cover your body and face with sunless solution via a machine. The first is the best way to get an even, streak-free result. The sunless tanner is also customized for each client's skin tone so that the most natural-looking color develops. In-booth spray-tanning sessions, such as those by Mystic Tan and California Tan, are less expensive but not as precise, though they do still hit hard-to-reach spots, like your back.

You don't have to head to a salon or spa to get a natural-looking golden glow. Today's at-home self-tanning products deliver amazing results. When I don't go to my sunless-tanning guru Anna Stankiewicz, owner of Suvara Spray Tan—whose celebrity clients include Jen Aniston, Blake Lively, and Maria Menounos—I, too, self-tan at home. Here, tips from Anna to do it like a pro:

1. If you're new to the world of self-tanning, start out slowly and look for goof-proof formulas that build color gradually over a few days.

2. Exfoliate your skin in the shower with a gentle scrub to create an even canvas for application.

3.   Apply self-tanner before bed. Sweat, tight clothes, and water are like kryptonite to sunless tanner. To ensure an even streak-free glow, sleep on it.

4.   Before you apply, rub body lotion onto your nails and cuticles, over your feet (ankles, balls, and heels), and across the outer and inner elbows—basically anywhere on your body that "creases." These areas tend to be drier so they absorb the product faster, resulting in uneven patches of color. A little lotion on these areas will act like a barrier and ensure even coverage.

5.   Always apply self-tanner in a circular motion to avoid streaks. Some new formulas come with application mitts that help spread the product evenly across your skin. Smooth extra on your tush and tummy. Golden dimples look less prominent and way more flattering than pasty white ones that scream cellulite.

6.   Do not bathe or shower for at least six hours after applying. That's the minimum amount of time needed for DHA (the active ingredient in sunless tanner) to sink in and work. If you get wet before then, color will not develop.

7.   After you apply self-tanner dust your entire body with talc-free baby powder. This will help set the product the same way face powder sets makeup. It banishes the stickiness and odor that's associated with sunless tanning and leaves you feeling fab with soft, touchable, baby-like skin.

8.   Do not apply deodorant or perfume when sunless tanning. They can alter the color of the tan.

9.   After applying, wait 10 minutes before dressing, and opt for loose-fitting dark clothes that won't be stained.

10.   Immediately wash hands with soap and water to avoid dark palms and fingers.

Feature Your Feet

Many times during the year, we can hide our feet in a way that we can hide few other parts of our body. Not feeling like they're especially sexy? A hot little shoe will take care of all that. But walking on the beach or by the pool calls for open-toe shoes, so you want your feet looking as pretty as they can be. To get ready for sandal season, I head to Jin Soon Nail Spa. Can't get there? Try these easy at-home pedicure tips:

Soak: A footbath softens dry skin so you can more easily slough it off. To do one, fill a basin or a tub with warm water, then add moisturizing olive oil and honey combined with muscle-calming Epsom salts. Let your feet soak for 10 minutes and they'll be prepped for exfoliations.

Smooth: Toward the end of your soak, put on textured mitts and then gently massage your feet with a gentle scrub. This will exfoliate your feet. For spots that are rough, try a pumice stone or foot file. And for callouses, you may need a heavy-duty tool that looks a little like a cheese grater but blasts through hardened dead layers immediately.

Hydrate: Use a moisturizer all over, even on the tops of your feet. Women tend to focus on the heels and balls of the feet, but moisturizer will help all around. A few nights a week, slather some on, then slip on thin cotton socks to let the ingredients sink in while you sleep (or just wear for an hour if you pre-

SALON SAFETY

Treating your toes to some pampering before your week at the beach? Heed this advice when heading to the nail spa:

✳ Bring your own tools to help reduce the risk of infection. If you don't have your own with you, make sure all metal implements have been sanitized and fresh files and buffers are used.

✳ Don't have your cuticles clipped or calluses razored. Even the tiniest of tears can lead to infection.

✳ Ask to make sure that footbath filters are cleaned after every client—that way your feet won't be exposed to a previous client's nails that are circulating in your soak.

fer to sleep sockless).

Shape: Trim your nails straight across, then file them with a fine-grade emery board. Push back your cuticles with an orange stick or washcloth, then use polish remover (one swipe each nail) to make them residue-free.

Polish: Separate your toes by lacing a twisted paper towel between them. After using a base coat, pick your color. Dunk the brush into the bottle just once for each nail and then cover each using three strokes—the first down the center with the bristle pushed so they fan out, then one on each side. (Too much polish can mean a gloppy finish, so you need only that one dunk.) Apply a second coat, then follow with a quick-dry clear top coat with UV absorbers; that will minimize fading. To perform any fixes, use a fine-tip paint or makeup brush, rather than a cotton swab ball (which can leave fuzzies in the wet paint).

Beat Body Blemishes

"Bacne," or back acne, is always a bummer, but it always feels worse during bikini season. Here are three reasons why those pesky pimples and painful cysts may be popping up and what you can do about it.

Hair products: The ingredients are designed to cling to hair, so they may stick to your skin, too, eventually plugging up pores. Wash and rinse your hair first, then soap up your body to get rid of any residue.

Sports bras: Tight-fitting clothes trap perspiration, which then mixes with bacteria, dirt, and oil on your skin, triggering a breakout. Swipe a salicylic acid-based towelette over acne-prone areas pre-gym. Shower immediately afterward.

Workouts: As you exercise, your adrenal glands pump out testosterone, which makes your skin produce more pore-clogging oil. Use an acne-fighting body wash on your back (one marked "for face" is fine) to exfoliate skin and eliminate the bacteria that cause blemishes.

PREVENT SUMMER PROBLEMS

THE PROBLEM	THE FIX
Swollen feet	Feet swell in the heat, so bring down inflammation with a 10-minute epsom salt soak. Also, elevate your feet as much as possible.
Tan lines	Fill in blanks with sunless-tanning products. But before you do, exfoliate skin to ensure an even application and flawless results. You can also blur tan lines temporarily with opaque body makeup.
Frizzy hair	Hydrate daily with conditioner to prevent strands from acting like a sponge (which will cause them to soak up moisture from humid air and make your hair unruly). Also add a frizz-fighting serum to your styling regimen.
Breakouts	Sweltering temps cause oil production to spike, and with a snug sports bra or bike helmet, it's the perfect recipe for clogged pores and pimples. To keep skin clear, exfoliate three times a week with a mild scrub and use a cleanser that contains glycolic or salicylic acid.
Dry hair	Days spent outdoors in the sun or swimming in salt or chlorinated water can take a toll—and create a vicious cycle: The more parched and straw-like the hair gets, the more prone to damage it becomes. Before going outside, spritz strands with a leave-in treatment that contains UV filters to help shield hair from the sun's harmful rays and conditions it, to treat dryness.
Chafing	Sweaty, heat-swollen feet can easily develop blisters when your shoes rub you the wrong way. The same is true for chafing with clothes on your thighs or other areas. To prevent it, dust on a body powder or swipe antiperspirant over your skin to minimize moisture while providing some slip.
Mottled chest skin	Sun exposure can lead to brown spots and broken capillaries that dot your décolletage. Mix in a few drops of a liquid highlighter with your foundation and smooth it over your chest to create an even-toned finish.
Spider veins	If you have only a few, you can use a concealer to cover them. But if you have a lot, try a body bronzer to help minimize the contrast between skin and veins. For a more permanent solution, ask your doctor about in-office treatments.

Pony Up
Your Hair

One of our favorite summer styles: A ponytail. These chic variations on the classic ponytail can be your go-to summer styles.

Bushy tailed: Mist the roots with a texturizing product. Next, finger-comb hair into a high ponytail, secure with an elastic, and loosen a few pieces at the crown. To thicken it, spritz with the same texturizer, then lightly tease with a brush.

Side winder: Run styling cream from roots to end, and comb it through to evenly distribute. Draw a side part; then form a tight, low ponytail and secure it with an elastic, leaving a small section in the front free. Next, take that loose piece and twist it into a long, taut coil. Wrap it around the base of your ponytail to hide the elastic, and lock the coil in place with bobby pins. Smooth more cream over the tail and hairline to tame flyaways.

Three-peat: Slick strands straight back, then gather only the top portion and anchor it with an elastic band, tight and flat against the back of your head. Repeat with the middle section, securing it at the center, and finally again with the bottom, fastening it at the nape of your neck. For extra sleekness, work a few drops of a smoother through the tail and gently over your hairline.

Dream weaver: To give hair grip, apply a beach spritzer, then create a deep side part. Weave a French braid along the hairline, using even amounts of hair for each section to maintain a uniform size all the way down. Pull everything into a low side ponytail and secure with an elastic band. Add luster with a light coating of shine spray.

Crown heights: Gather all your hair, except for the top section—which you can push aside for now—and tie it into a low ponytail. Apply a root booster at the crown, then backcomb the area until you've created a three-inch "cushion." Smooth the top section over the teased area, then brush it down and over the first ponytail and secure with a second elastic. Hide the band by winding a piece from the tail around it and fasten with a bobby pin. Lock the style in place with hairspray.

Stay Cool

Of course, we want you to sweat hard when you're working out, but sometimes, we sweat when we least want to. In fact, about 20 percent of people say they perspire too much (3 percent of people have a condition called hyperhidrosis, meaning that they sweat so much that it interferes with their lives). Here, some tips for taking the ire out of perspiring.

Rethink your wardrobe: Choose natural, breathable fabrics like linen and cotton in light colors (dark colors absorb more sun). Wear loose layers to keep air flowing; you can also peel off layers as you start sweating. If you sweat a lot under your arms or in between your legs, try moisture-wicking tees and underwear.

Change antiperspirants: Trade up to a clinical-strength formula, which, compared with regular ones, contains a higher percentage of aluminum zirconium tetrachlorohydrex, an effective over-the-counter sweat-stopper. Antiperspirant does a better job of blocking sweat glands if you put it on in the evening (when most people perspire less), so swipe it on before bed. Then reapply in the morning for extra protection.

Get an R$_x$: If OTC options aren't working for you, ask a dermatologist about Drysol or Hypercare, which have a higher percentage of aluminum chloride. That makes them stronger but also more likely to irritate skin. In severe cases, an oral drug may help.

Invest in long-term help: Botox is known as a wrinkle-smoother, but since 2004, it's been FDA-approved to combat sweat, too. It interferes with the nerves that stimulate sweat glands and can cut perspiration by more than 75 percent for up to seven months. You'll need treatments a few times a year to keep sweat at bay, but I think the cost is worth it. I get Botox under my arms, and it has changed my life. Hello, silk blouses!

Be On Guard

Summer should be fun, but sometimes, our anything-goes attitude can get us into a little trouble. Here, three small but important summer safety tips:

Watch the booze. Not only are those yummy piña coladas and daiquiris loaded with calories, the alcohol can make you a little relaxed and less diligent about applying and reapplying sunscreen. So drink with care.

Don't linger in a wet suit. That will help you avoid skin irritation and yeast infections. Change into dry clothes when you're done splashing around.

Don't walk all day in flips. Flip-flops are easy, but because of that, they can also cause you some foot problems. According to research published in the *Journal of the American Podiatric Medical Association*, flip-flops can change your gait and lead to ankle sprains and plantar fasciitis (inflammation of the tissue connecting your heel to your toes). And you can even widen your feet if you wear them too much, since the lack of support under your sole causes your foot to splay out and can loosen the soft tissue over time. Experts recommend walking no more than one hour a day in them.

Most Importantly: Protect Your Skin!

Looking beautiful isn't just about maximizing your look; it's also about knowing how to protect your skin from harmful rays. While we're all for loving the sun, you have to remember that sun damage can not only lead to health problems (it's the leading cause of skin cancer), but is also what ages our skin quickly—and takes away that youthful glow. To shield your skin, use sunscreen daily.

Apply It Right

WATCH THE CLOCK

Put on sunscreen at least 30 minutes before stepping outdoors. "It takes that long for the protective ingredients to bind to skin," says Vivian Bucay, M.D., a dermatologist in San Antonio. To avoid missing spots, smooth it on as evenly as possible prior to getting dressed. I find that applying it naked in front of the mirror is the best way to ensure you're fully covered.

LAY IT ON THICK

To borrow from an old adage, an ounce of sunscreen really is worth a pound of cure. On beach days, coat your body entirely with at least that much (fill a shot glass to be sure you're using enough), saving 1 teaspoon for your face, ears, and neck. Using a spray? "You have to spritz liberally," says Bucay. "A fine mist isn't going to cover you fully." Her recommendation: Time how long it takes to spray one ounce into a shot glass, then spritz it on your body for at least that long. Don't forget to put sunscreen on the tips of your ears and on the tops of your feet. These spots are especially painful when burned.

REPEAT, REPEAT, REPEAT

Sunscreen's protective power is strongest when it's fairly fresh on your skin, so apply it often. To stay on schedule, set your phone timer to go off every two hours (more often if you're sweating, soaking, or drying off with a towel), and then slather on another ounce.

Label Lowdown

In the past, sunscreens labeled "broad-spectrum" were able to claim a high SPF (the measure of how well they protect against "burning" UVB rays) but could still have wimpy protection against "aging" UVA rays. (Sobering statistic: More than 95 percent of the rays we're exposed to are UVA and, compared with UVB rays, they generate far more free radicals that lead to wrinkles and brown spots.) Now products have to contain proportional protection in order to be labeled broad-spectrum. "That means the greater a sunscreen's SPF, the more protection it provides against both UVA and UVB damage," explains Arielle N.B. Kauvar, M.D., clinical professor of dermatology at New York University School of Medicine. Sunscreens with SPF less than 15 are no longer permitted to claim they offer broad-spectrum protection and are now required to have a warning that they help prevent sunburn only; those with higher SPFs are allowed to be labeled broad-spectrum and state that they help guard against premature skin aging and skin cancer.

NO "WATERPROOF," "SWEATPROOF," OR "SUNBLOCK" CLAIMS

These terms have been eliminated because they overstate the effectiveness of sunscreens, giving users a false sense of security. Instead, those that pass certain tests are labeled "water resistant" and are required to list the amount of time you can expect to get the protection promised on the bottle while swimming and sweating—either 40 or 80 minutes.

Always read the fine print to ensure you're getting grade-A UVA protection. Check under "active ingredients" for the most effective UVA shields, including a combo of avobenzone and octocrylene (sometimes marketed under the brand names Helioplex and AvoTriplex); ecamsule (aka Mexoryl SX); and zinc oxide. (Or choose one of the sunscreens mentioned here, which all fit the bill.) And no matter what the label implies, always apply a fresh coat every two hours—or more frequently if you're swimming or perspiring heavily.

Stay-Safe Strategies

✳ **Don't skip days.** Sunscreen should be applied year-round, rain or shine: UVB rays may be stronger during the summer, but UVA shines down on us day in and day out, says New York University's Kauvar.

✳ **Do opt for an SPF 30 (or higher).** SPF 15 shields about 93 percent of UVB light; SPF 30 buffers 97 percent. But those percentages pertain to laboratory settings, not real life—which is why derms recommend hedging your bets with higher-SPF screens. "Studies also show that people use one-third to one-half of the amount they need to get the SPF on the bottle," says Steven Q. Wang, M.D., director of dermatologic surgery at Memorial Sloan-Kettering Cancer Center in Basking Ridge, NJ, and a member of the Skin Cancer Foundation's photobiology committee. "So while the label may say SPF 30, you're getting closer to SPF 15 or 10." Aim even higher if you're particularly sun-vulnerable—for instance, if you're on oral or topical medications like antibiotics, birth control pills, hormone therapy, antidepressants, retinoids, or natural remedies like St. John's wort; or if you suffer from an autoimmune disease like lupus.

✳ **Don't rely only on SPF.** Wearing hats, sunglasses, and clothing with built-in protection are musts, says Wang, as is shunning the sun between the hours of 10 a.m. and 4 p.m.—when burning rays are out in force. Staying in the shade reduces UV exposure by as much as 50 percent.

LOVE THE SUN, BUT DON'T BATHE IN IT

We love everything that summer stands for, and there's nothing that feels quite as invigorating and healing as spending some time out in the sun. But as we all know by now, just because it feels good doesn't mean it is good. In fact, 90 percent of skin cancers are caused by the sun's ultraviolet rays. Those rays are more intense in the summer, but we should all be in the habit of protecting our skin from the sun's damaging rays year round—for the health concerns foremost, but also because sun damage is one of the things that ages our skin and causes us to lose our glow.

Skin Cancer by the Numbers

More than 2 million people will be diagnosed with the disease this year. Here's how to avoid being one of them.

90

Percent of skin cancers caused by the sun's ultraviolet rays. The shorter UVB rays are more intense in the summer, but the longer UVA rays remain constant year-round—hence the need to apply sunscreen every day, rain or shine. Both types of UV light can cause skin cancer, but "A" rays are also responsible for wrinkles, brown spots, and other signs of skin aging. Don't count on overcast skies to protect you, either, as 80 percent of UV penetrates haze, fog, and light clouds. "Unless it's so dark outside that you need a flashlight to see, you should be wearing sunscreen," says Doris J. Day, M.D., clinical associate professor of dermatology at New York University Langone Medical Center.

30

Minimum SPF you should be using. To be effective against both UVA and UVB, your sunscreen must provide broad-spectrum protection (it will say so on the label).

1 OUNCE

The amount of sunscreen you should apply to your entire body to get the SPF promised on the label. Research shows the average person applies just one-quarter to one-half of that amount. "That means an SPF 30 is really an SPF 15 or 7," says Steven Q. Wang, M.D., director of dermatologic surgery and dermatology at Memorial Sloan-Kettering Cancer Center.

15 Minutes

The length of time before going outside that you should apply sunscreen; this will give your skin enough time to absorb the protective ingredients. "Smooth it on as evenly as possible before getting dressed to avoid missing spots, especially areas near clothing edges that may move with exercise," says Arielle Kauvar, M.D., clinical professor of dermatology at New York University Langone Medical Center.

21

Percent less likely that coffee drinkers who have more than three cups a day are to develop basal cell carcinoma (BCC) than those who rarely enjoy a cup, according to a recent study in Cancer Research. Most common in folks older than 55, BCC has more than doubled in younger women over the past 30 years. Prefer tea? Research shows that the green variety heals rough pre-cancerous patches known as actinic keratosis (AK), while black tea with lemon markedly reduced the risk of squamous cell carcinoma (SCC).

100

Number of minutes of unprotected sun exposure it takes to suppress your immune system by 50 percent. This lowering of the body's defenses raises your risk of skin cancer.

2 HOURS

How frequently you need to reapply sunscreen. If you're swimming or sweating excessively, slather on more even sooner—one study in the journal *Clinics in Dermatology* showed that perspiration makes skin more prone to burning.

10 A.M. to 2 P.M.

The peak hours of UV light. If you can't avoid outdoor activities during this time, Wang advises dressing defensively, which includes wearing a long-sleeve shirt, a wide-brim hat, wraparound sunglasses, and covered shoes. To increase clothing's SPF to 30, there are SPF laundry additives you can toss into your wash.

47

Percent of lifetime sun exposure acquired by age 40. The take-home message: It's never too late to start wearing sunscreen. One recent study of adults showed that a decade of wearing sunscreen cut their likelihood of developing melanoma, the most dangerous form of skin cancer, in half; other research found that daily use led to fewer AKs, as well as less BCC and SCC, the most common forms of the disease. "It's similar to when people stop smoking cigarettes," says Kauvar. "Their risk of lung cancer diminishes over time."

3 in 10

Number of melanomas that begin in moles. If one looks suspicious (tip-offs include a change in size, shape, or color), be sure to tell your derm ASAP. A big don't: relying on smartphone apps to diagnose skin lesions. In a new study published in *JAMA Dermatology*, three out of four apps incorrectly classified at least 30 percent of melanomas as not dangerous. While most cancer-spotting apps rely on computer algorithms to predict if moles are malignant, cancer doesn't always fit neatly into most equations, say researchers.

40-60

Percent less UV exposure you'll receive when you seek the shade, according to Richard Grant, PhD., a professor of agronomy at Purdue University.

EIGHT-FOLD

Increase in melanoma rates among women younger than 40 over the past 40 years, a surge that may correspond to the skyrocketing rates of indoor tanning among young adults. You don't have to be a regular at the fake 'n' bake to raise your risk of developing melanoma: It takes only one session to up your odds by 20 percent. Not surprisingly, the International Agency for Research on Cancer has elevated the use of tanning beds—which is also responsible for 170,000 new cases of BCC and SCC annually—to the highest possible cancer-risk category. To help kick the habit (but not the bronze hue), switch to sunless tanner. In one study, 73 percent of people decreased indoor tanning when they began using it. DIY tanners also tend to use more sunscreen.

26

Percent of women who've had a skin exam by a dermatologist. "Early detection is the best chance for cure," says Kauvar, who recommends yearly exams of your birthday suit. Consider this: When melanoma is caught before it penetrates the skin, the five-year survival rate is 100 percent; once it spreads to other parts of the body, survival rates drop to as low as 16 percent. Since getting to know your own skin will help you identify any new or changing areas, monthly self-checks are also in order.

1

Number of people who die from melanoma every hour.

50

Percent reduction in melanoma when people ate a Mediterranean-style diet, which includes lots of fruits and vegetables, as well as olive oil and fish. The findings, which were published in the International Journal of Epidemiology, are likely the result of the diet's abundant supply of antioxidants, substances that help protect against cellular damage caused by UV radiation. Another reason to go fish: Regularly eating omega-3-fatty-acid- rich varieties like salmon, mackerel, and trout not only kept AKs at bay in one *American Journal of Clinical Nutrition* study, but it also led to less immune system suppression in another—which could help stave off skin cancer.

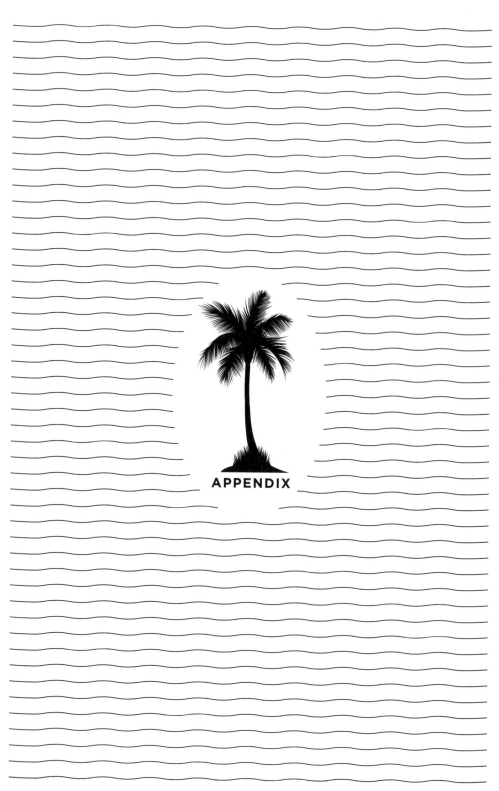

APPENDIX

Your
Bikini Body
Diet
DAILY LOG

One thing I and many of my friends in the health and fitness industry have noticed: We get better results when we keep track of what we do each day. I don't mean we make a mental note of what we ate or which workout we did. I mean we make a written note.

A formal food and workout log is a fantastic way to ensure that you stay on track toward your goals. You'll always know what you ate. You'll always know which workout you did. Keeping tabs like this makes it easier for you to stay the course, eat the right foods, and never miss a workout. Think about it this way: If you always eat right and never miss a workout, *it's impossible to fail*. The math is that simple!

Plus, I encourage you to keep track of things like how well you slept and what your energy level is. Why? As you make your way through the Bikini Body Diet, you'll be able to spot trends. For example: A week of lousy sleep will knock down your energy levels, spiking food cravings. Use this log to see how well you're doing and what tweaks may boost results.

The following is eight daily log pages. Make photocopies for the remainder of the program—and for however long you want to keep track of your daily progress. It's a healthy habit you can keep for the rest of your life. Trust me, do this and incorporate the Bikini Body Diet BEACH foods and you'll be strutting your stuff in a bikini in no time.

Your Bikini Body Diet DAILY LOG

TODAY'S MEALS   DATE _____

Breakfast _____

_____

_____

Lunch _____

_____

_____

Dinner _____

_____

_____

How many glasses of water did I drink today?

1 2 3 4 5 6 7 8 MORE?

What supplements did I take today?

_____

My sleep quality last night was...   **1 2 3 4 5 6 7 8 9 10**
                                Lousy   *Dreamy*

My energy level today was...   **1 2 3 4 5 6 7 8 9 10**
                          Nonexistent   *Off the charts*

I did the following workout today:

_____

_____

_____

Positive changes I noticed today:

_____

_____

_____

Your Bikini Body Diet DAILY LOG

_____
DATE

TODAY'S MEALS

Breakfast _____
_____
_____

Lunch _____
_____
_____

Dinner _____
_____
_____

How many glasses of water did I drink today?

  1 2 3 4 5 6 7 8 MORE?

What supplements did I take today?

_____

My sleep quality last night was... **1 2 3 4 5 6 7 8 9 10**
  Lousy   *Dreamy*

My energy level today was... **1 2 3 4 5 6 7 8 9 10**
  Nonexistent   *Off the charts*

I did the following workout today:

_____
_____
_____

Positive changes I noticed today:

_____
_____
_____

Your Bikini Body Diet DAILY LOG

TODAY'S MEALS

DATE _____

Breakfast _____
_____
_____
_____

Lunch _____
_____
_____
_____

Dinner _____
_____
_____

How many glasses of water did I drink today?

1 2 3 4 5 6 7 8 MORE?

What supplements did I take today?

_____

My sleep quality last night was... **1 2 3 4 5 6 7 8 9 10**
Lousy   *Dreamy*

My energy level today was... **1 2 3 4 5 6 7 8 9 10**
Nonexistent   *Off the charts*

I did the following workout today:

_____
_____
_____

Positive changes I noticed today:

_____
_____
_____

Your Bikini Body Diet DAILY LOG

DATE

TODAY'S MEALS

Breakfast_____

_____

_____

Lunch _____

_____

_____

Dinner_____

_____

_____

How many glasses of water did I drink today?

1   2   3   4   5   6   7   8   MORE?

What supplements did I take today?

_____

My sleep quality last night was... **1   2   3   4   5   6   7   8   9   10**
Lousy   *Dreamy*

My energy level today was... **1   2   3   4   5   6   7   8   9   10**
Nonexistent   *Off the charts*

I did the following workout today:

_____

_____

_____

Positive changes I noticed today:

_____

_____

_____

Your Bikini Body Diet DAILY LOG

TODAY'S MEALS **DATE**

Breakfast_____
_____
_____

Lunch _____
_____
_____

Dinner_____
_____
_____

How many glasses of water did I drink today?

1 2 3 4 5 6 7 8 MORE?

What supplements did I take today?

_____

My sleep quality last night was... **1 2 3 4 5 6 7 8 9 10**
Lousy   *Dreamy*

My energy level today was... **1 2 3 4 5 6 7 8 9 10**
Nonexistent   *Off the charts*

I did the following workout today:

_____
_____
_____

Positive changes I noticed today:

_____
_____
_____

Your Bikini Body Diet DAILY LOG

TODAY'S MEALS

Breakfast _____
_____
_____

Lunch _____
_____
_____

Dinner _____
_____
_____

How many glasses of water did I drink today?

1 2 3 4 5 6 7 8 MORE?

What supplements did I take today?

_____

My sleep quality last night was... **1 2 3 4 5 6 7 8 9 10**
                                     Lousy   _Dreamy_

My energy level today was... **1 2 3 4 5 6 7 8 9 10**
                              Nonexistent   _Off the charts_

I did the following workout today:

_____
_____
_____

Positive changes I noticed today:

_____
_____
_____

Your Bikini Body Diet DAILY LOG

TODAY'S MEALS

DATE _____

Breakfast _____
_____
_____

Lunch _____
_____
_____

Dinner _____
_____
_____

How many glasses of water did I drink today?

1 2 3 4 5 6 7 8 MORE?

What supplements did I take today?

_____

My sleep quality last night was... **1 2 3 4 5 6 7 8 9 10**
                                          Lousy   *Dreamy*

My energy level today was... **1 2 3 4 5 6 7 8 9 10**
                                  Nonexistent   *Off the charts*

I did the following workout today:

_____
_____
_____

Positive changes I noticed today:

_____
_____
_____

Your Bikini Body Diet DAILY LOG

DATE _____

TODAY'S MEALS

Breakfast _____

_____

_____

Lunch _____

_____

_____

Dinner _____

_____

_____

How many glasses of water did I drink today?

1 2 3 4 5 6 7 8 MORE?

What supplements did I take today?

_____

My sleep quality last night was... **1 2 3 4 5 6 7 8 9 10**
Lousy   *Dreamy*

My energy level today was... **1 2 3 4 5 6 7 8 9 10**
Nonexistent   *Off the charts*

I did the following workout today:

_____

_____

_____

Positive changes I noticed today:

_____

_____

_____

271

Index

A

B

INDEX